PICTURE BOOK OF
COLORFUL
BIRDS

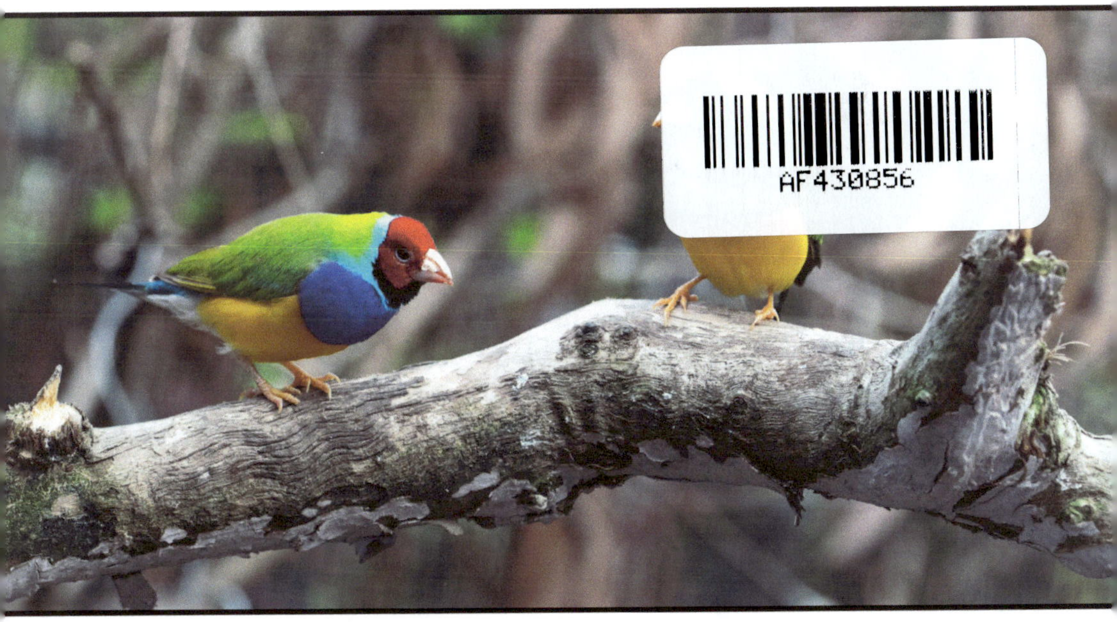

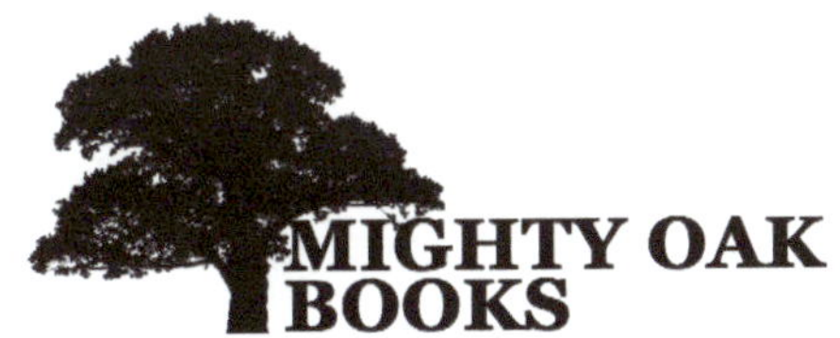

MIGHTY OAK BOOKS

American Goldfinch

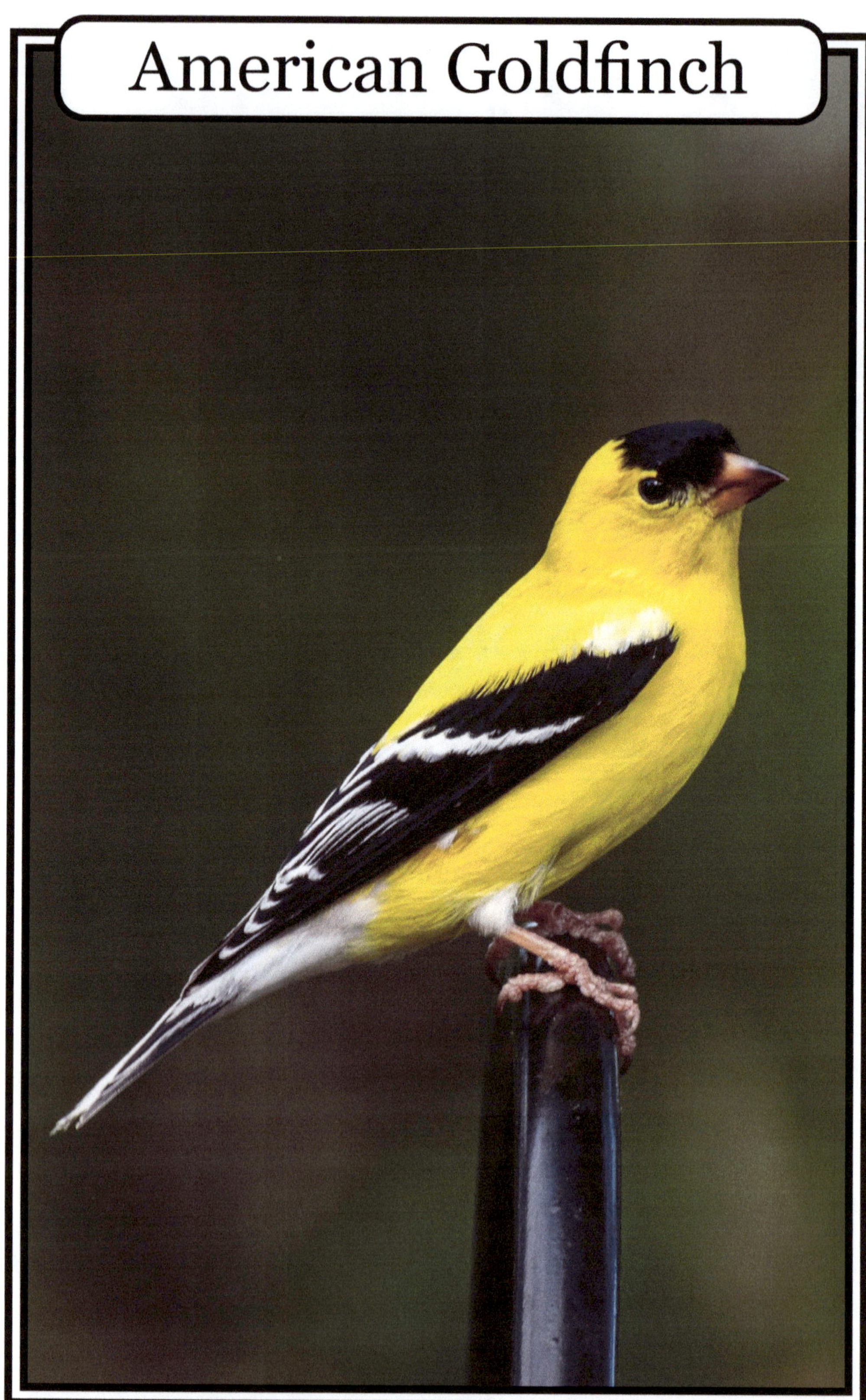

Jambu Fruit Dove

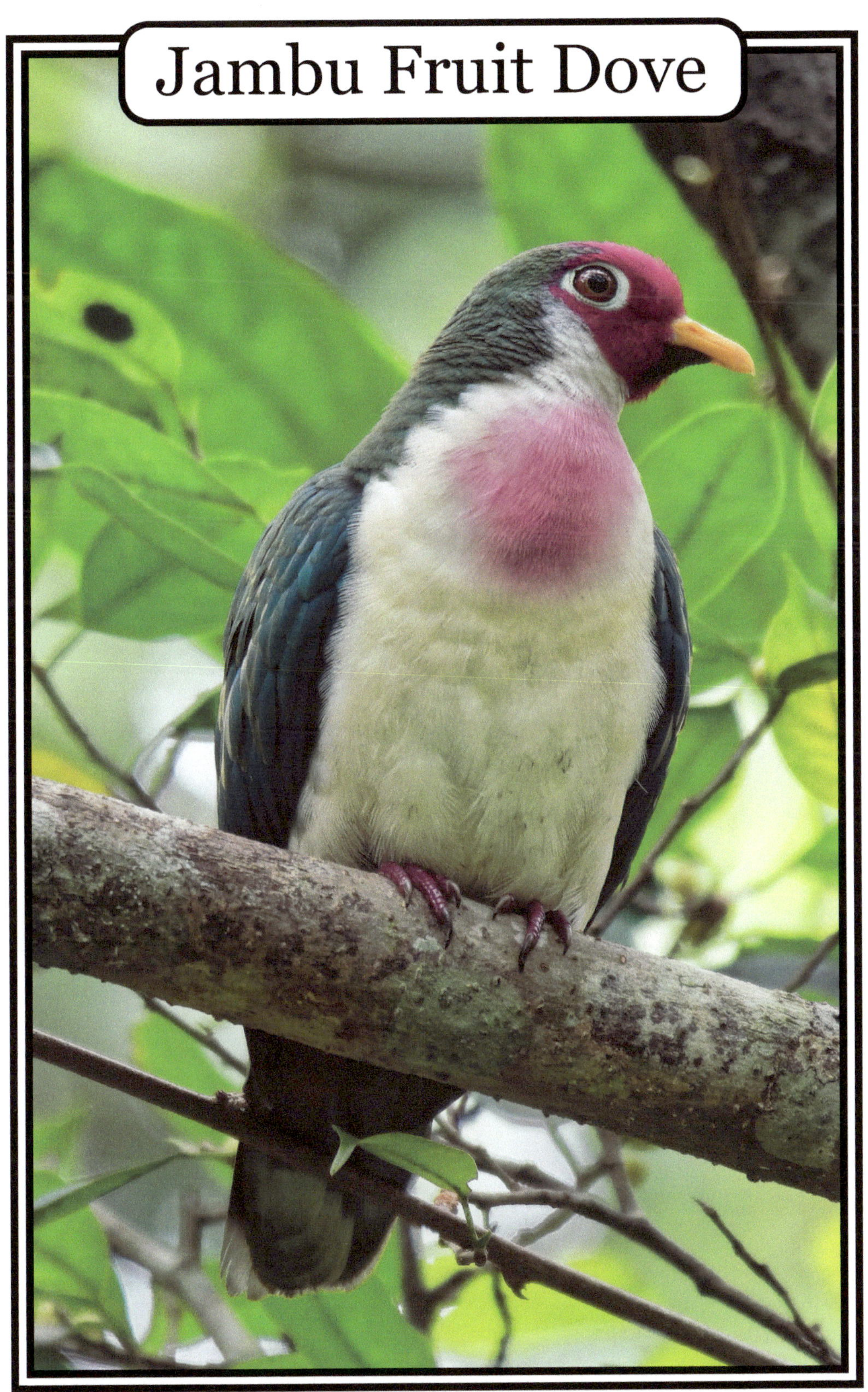

European Bee-Eater

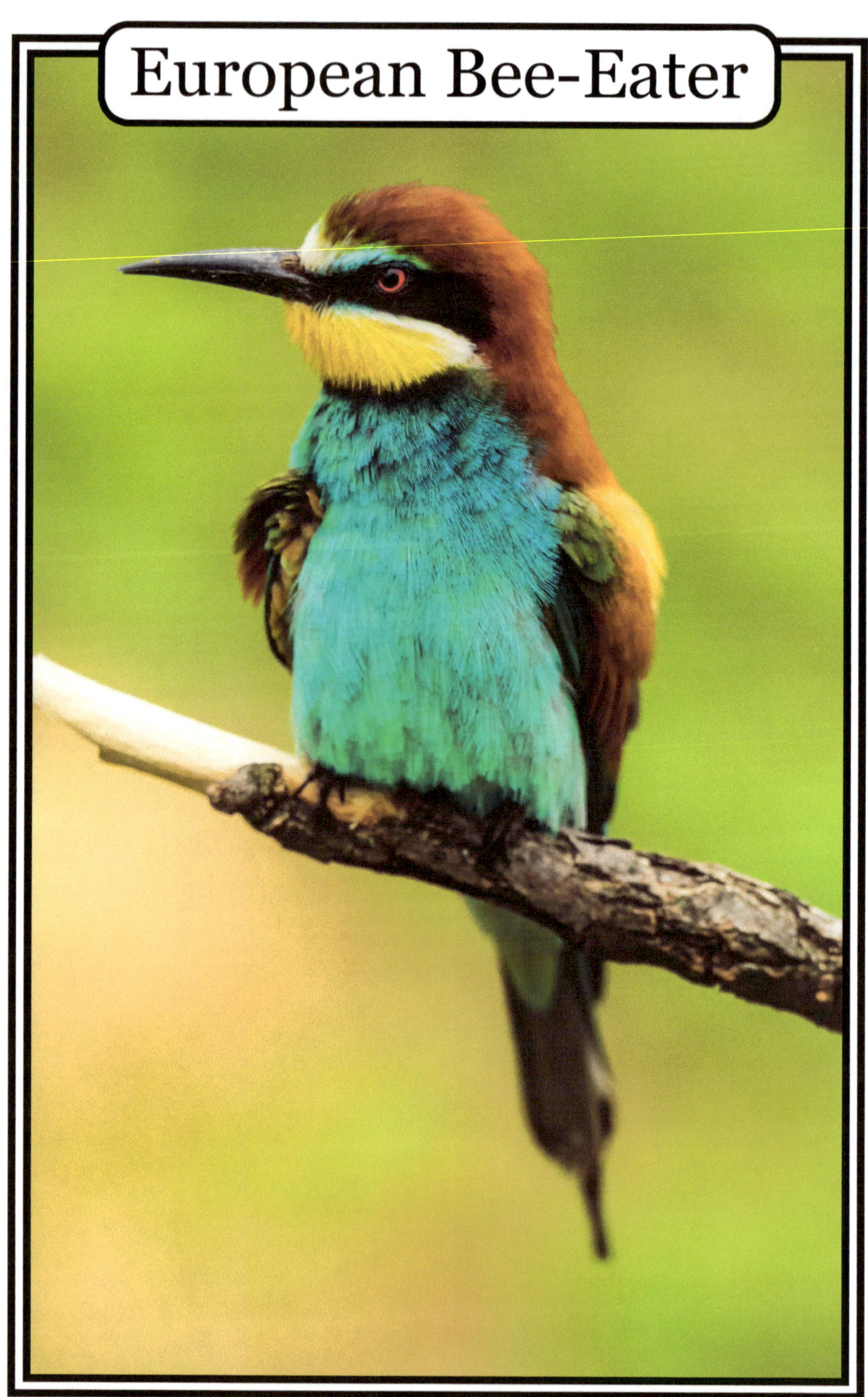

Flamingo

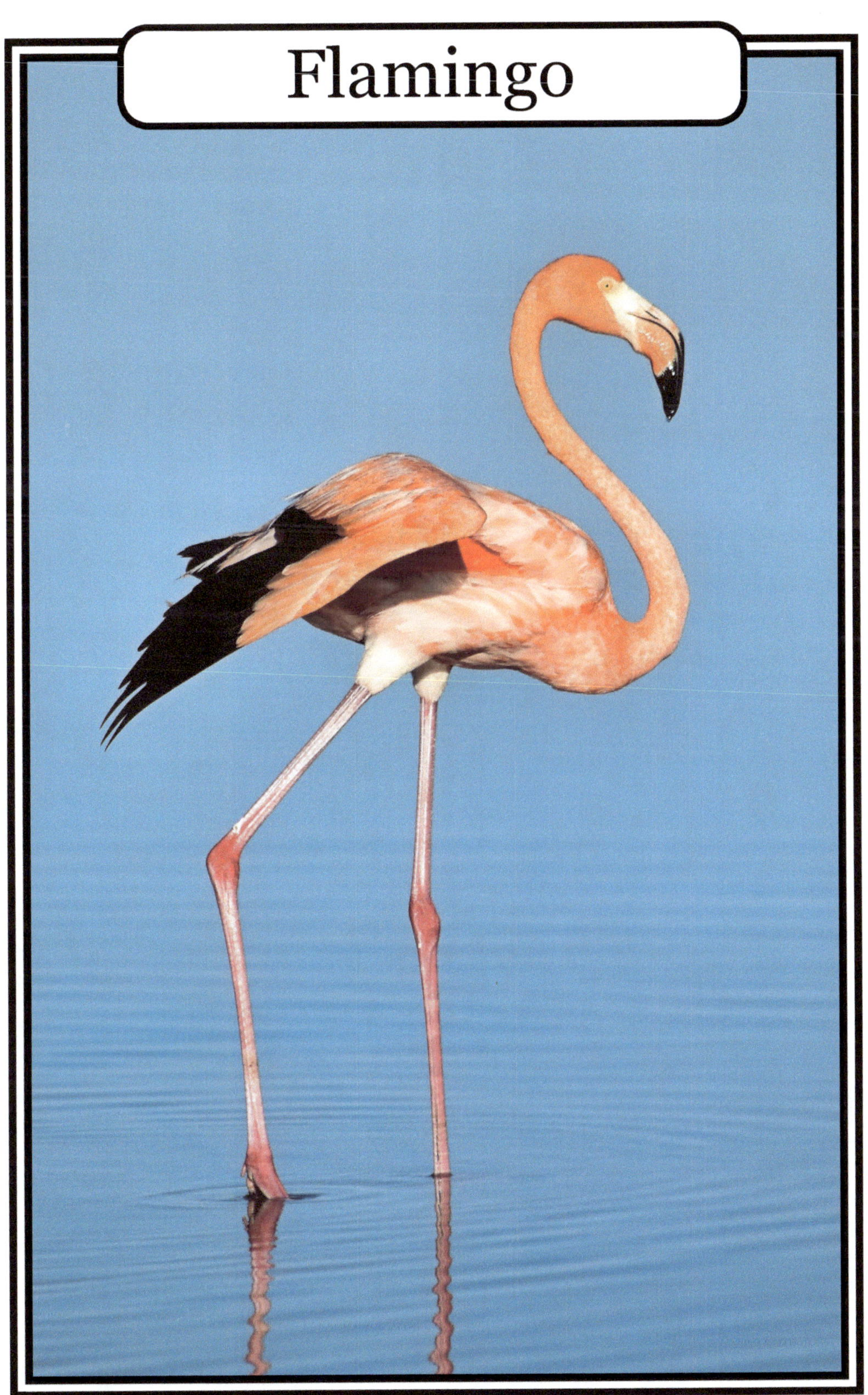

Common Kingfisher

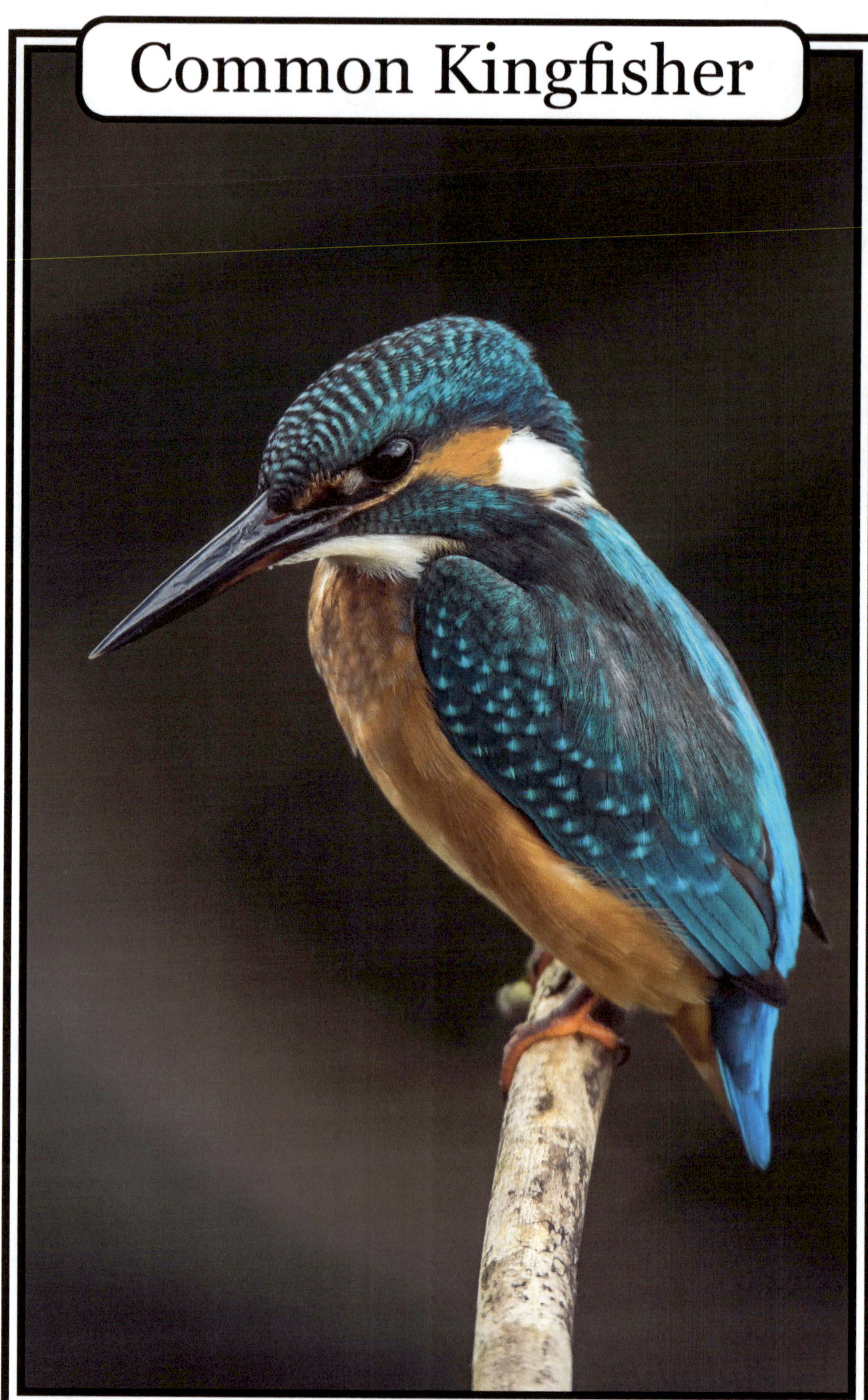

Blue Jay

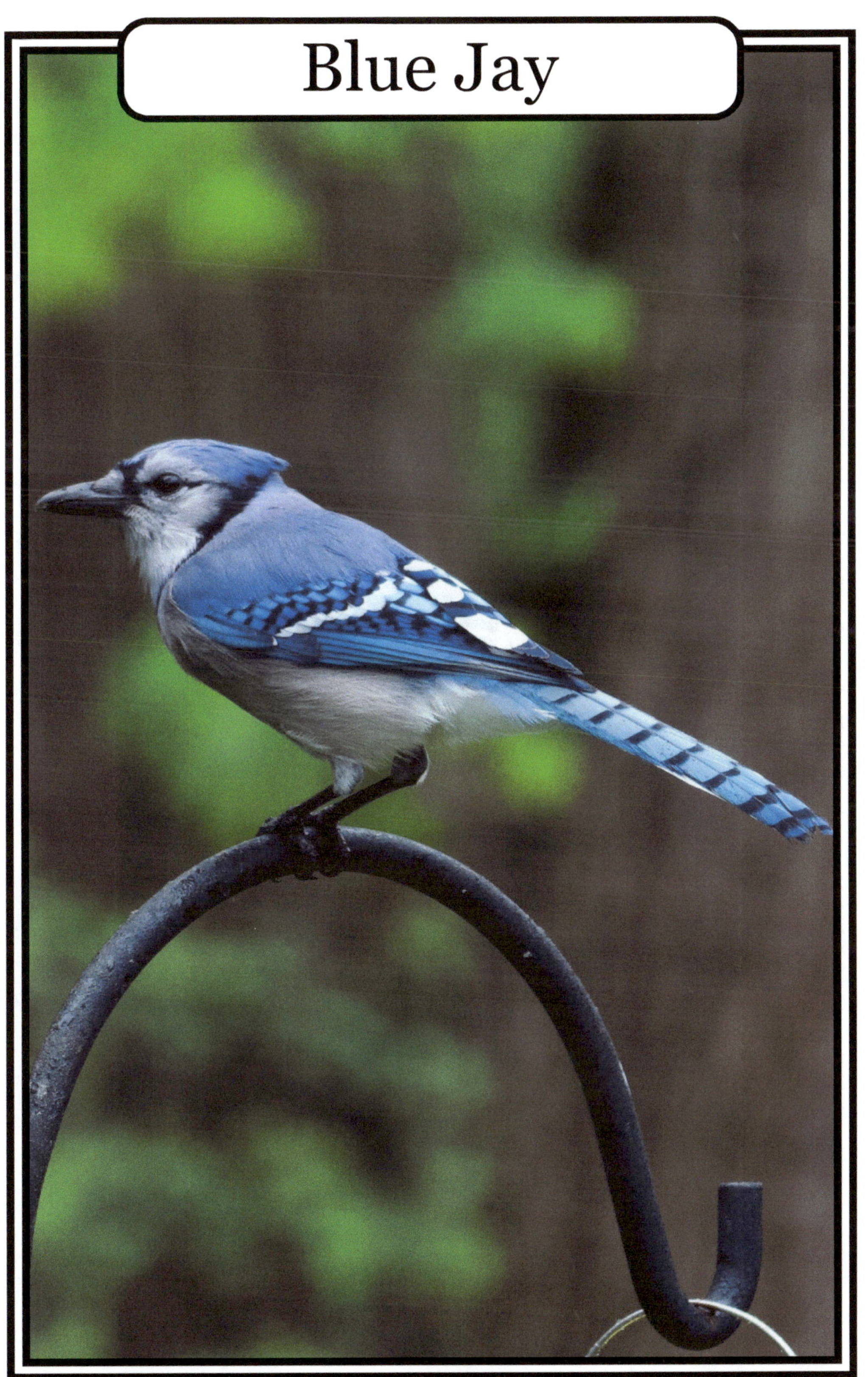

Cardinal

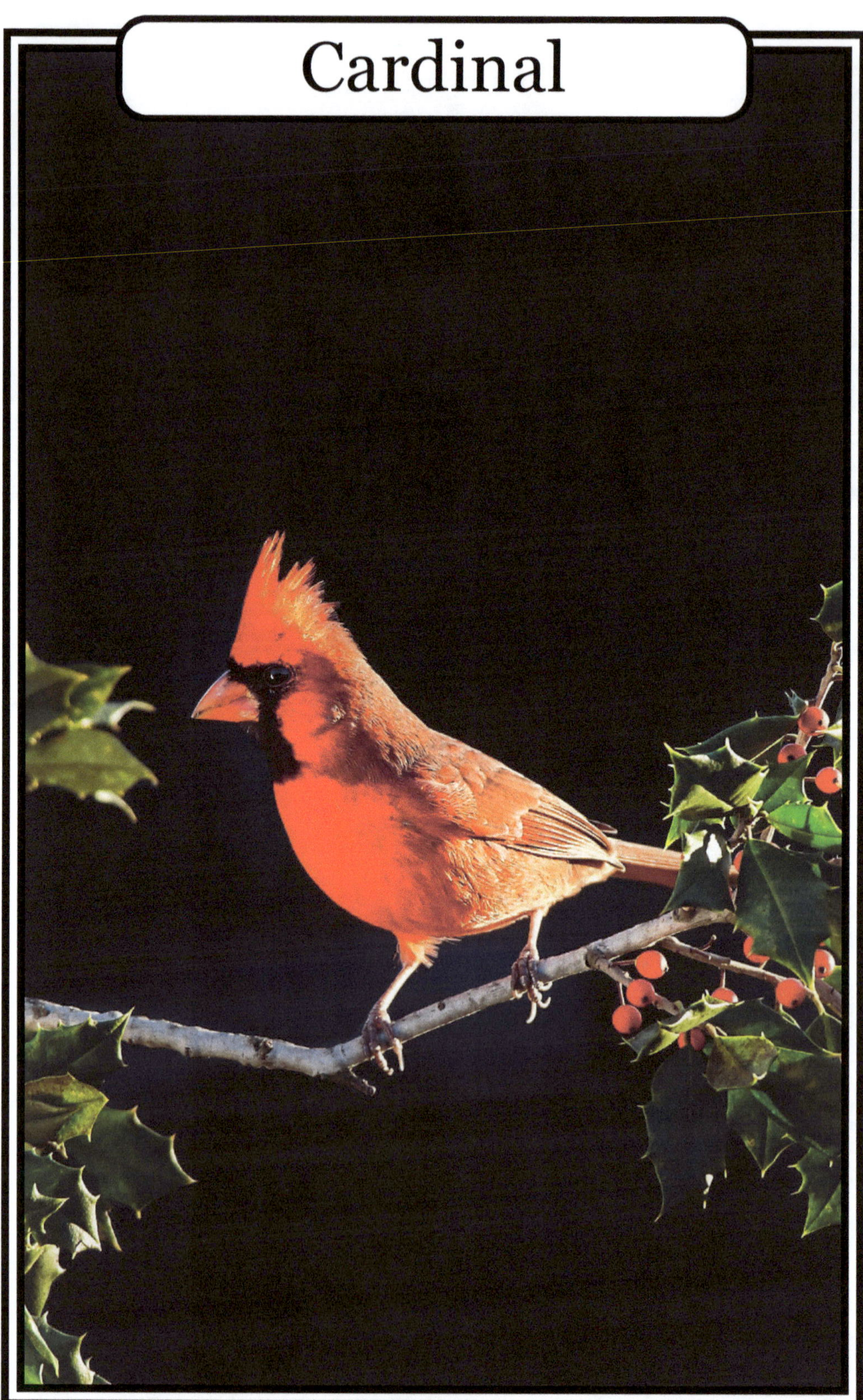

Baltimore Oriole

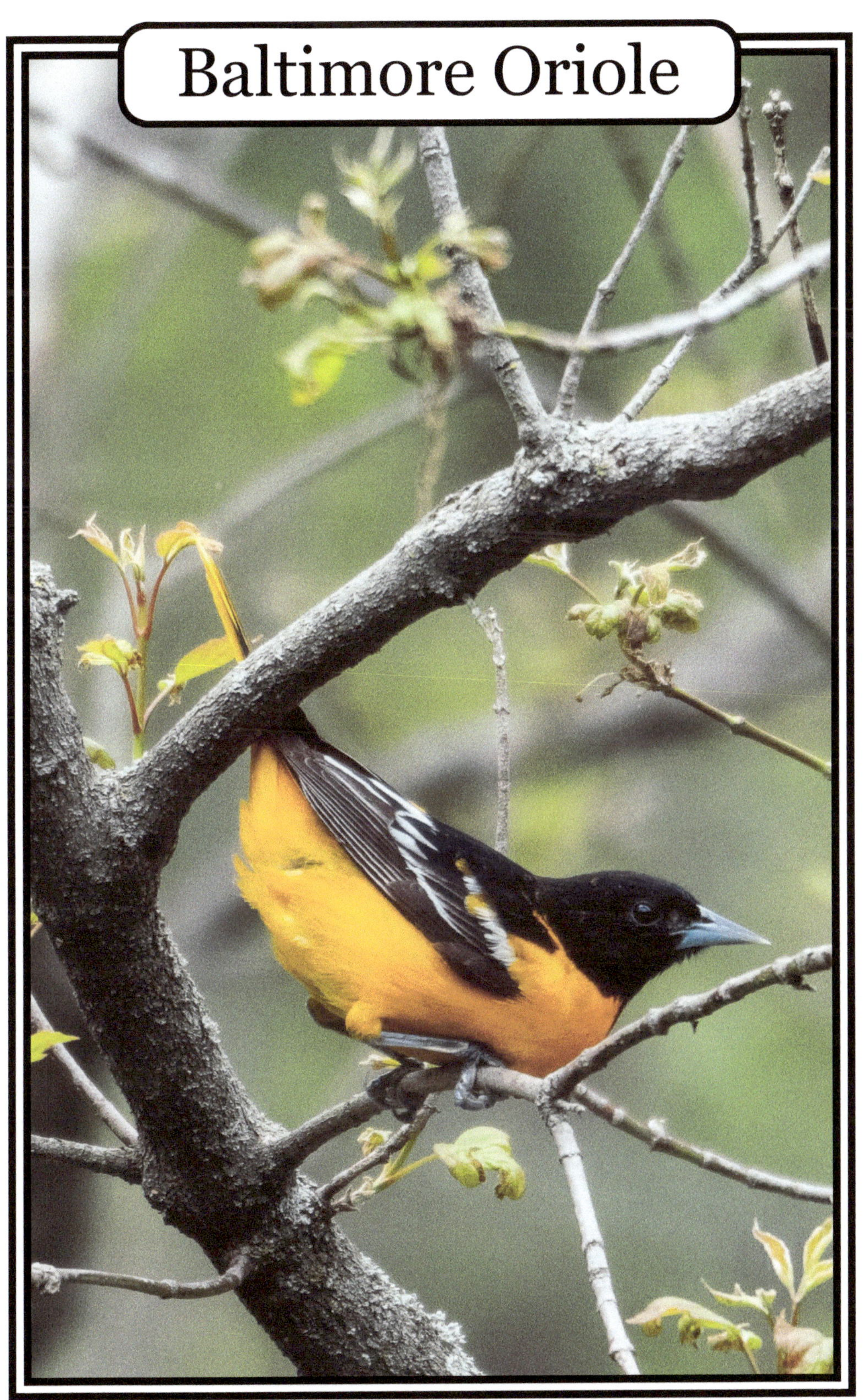

Rainbow-Billed Toucan

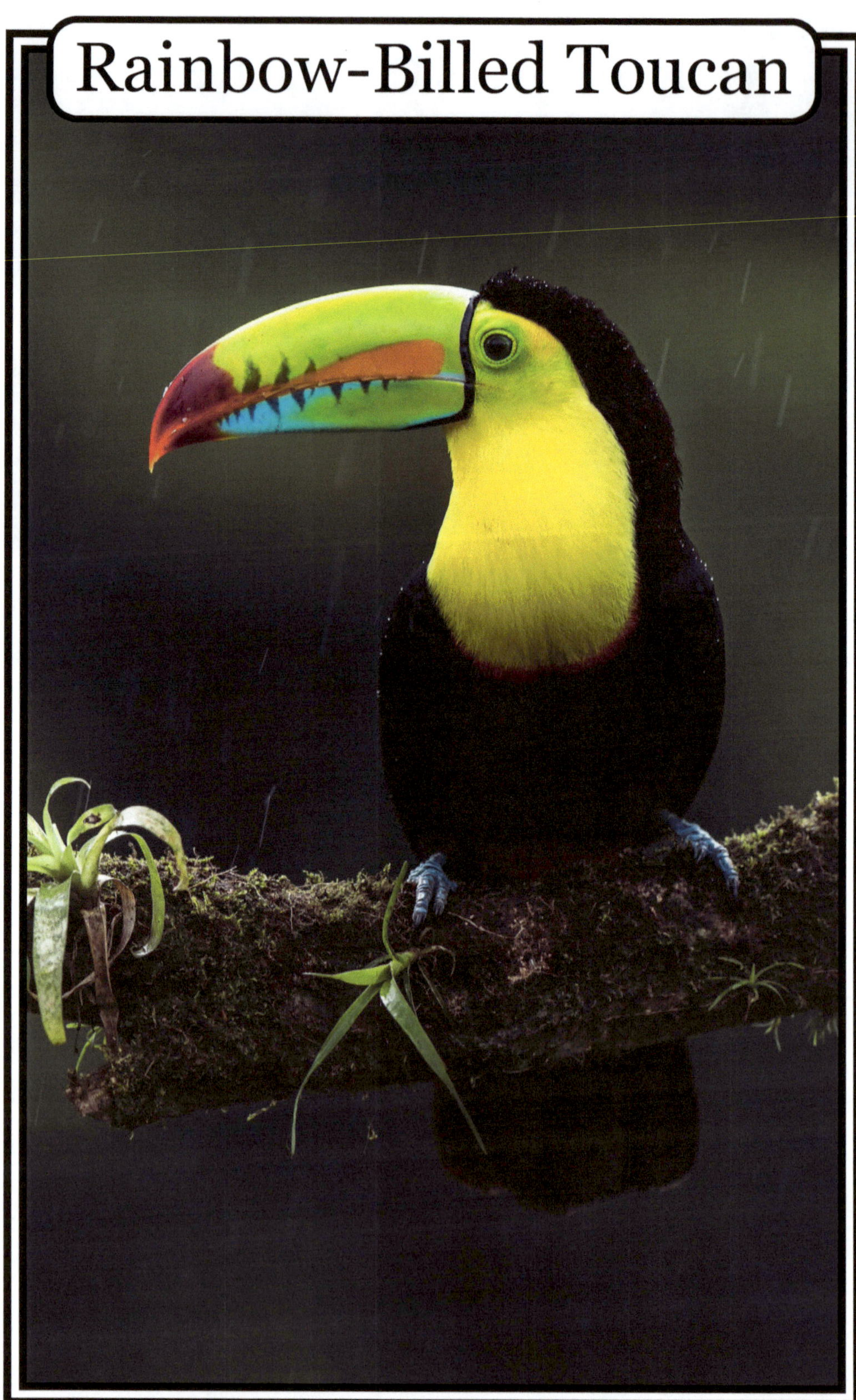

Violetear Hummingbird

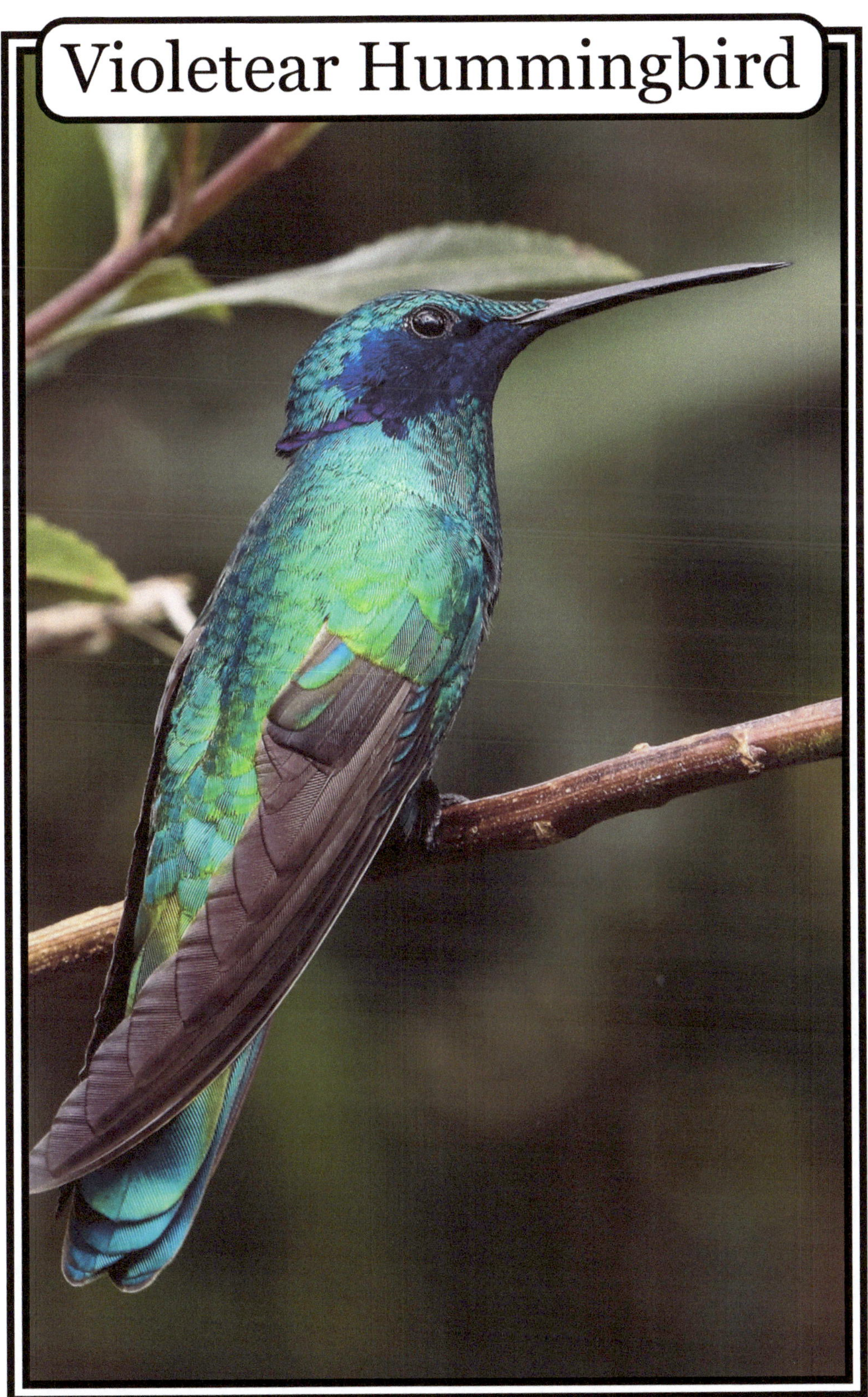

Blue-and-Yellow Macaw

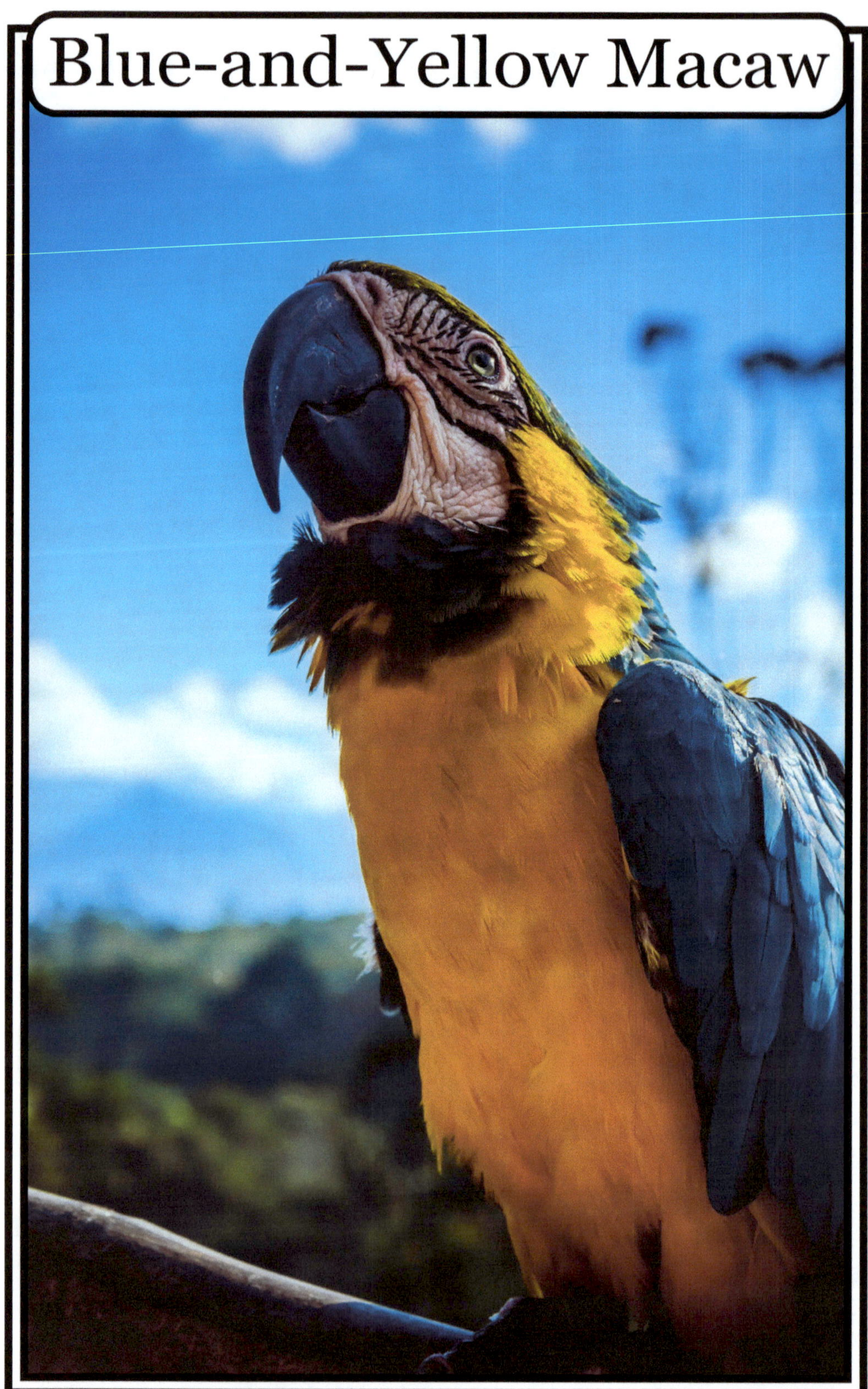

Cockatiel

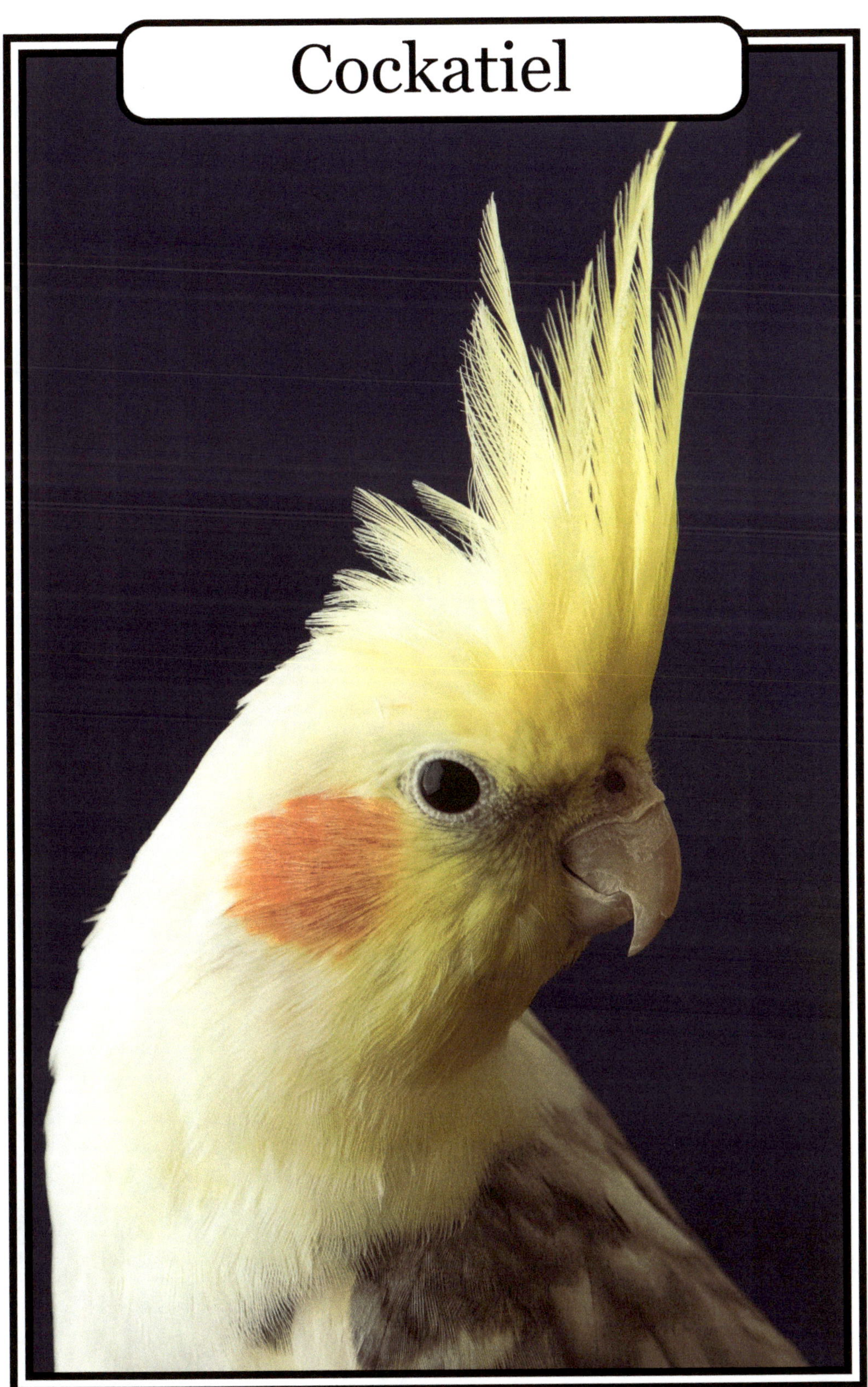

Dusky Lory

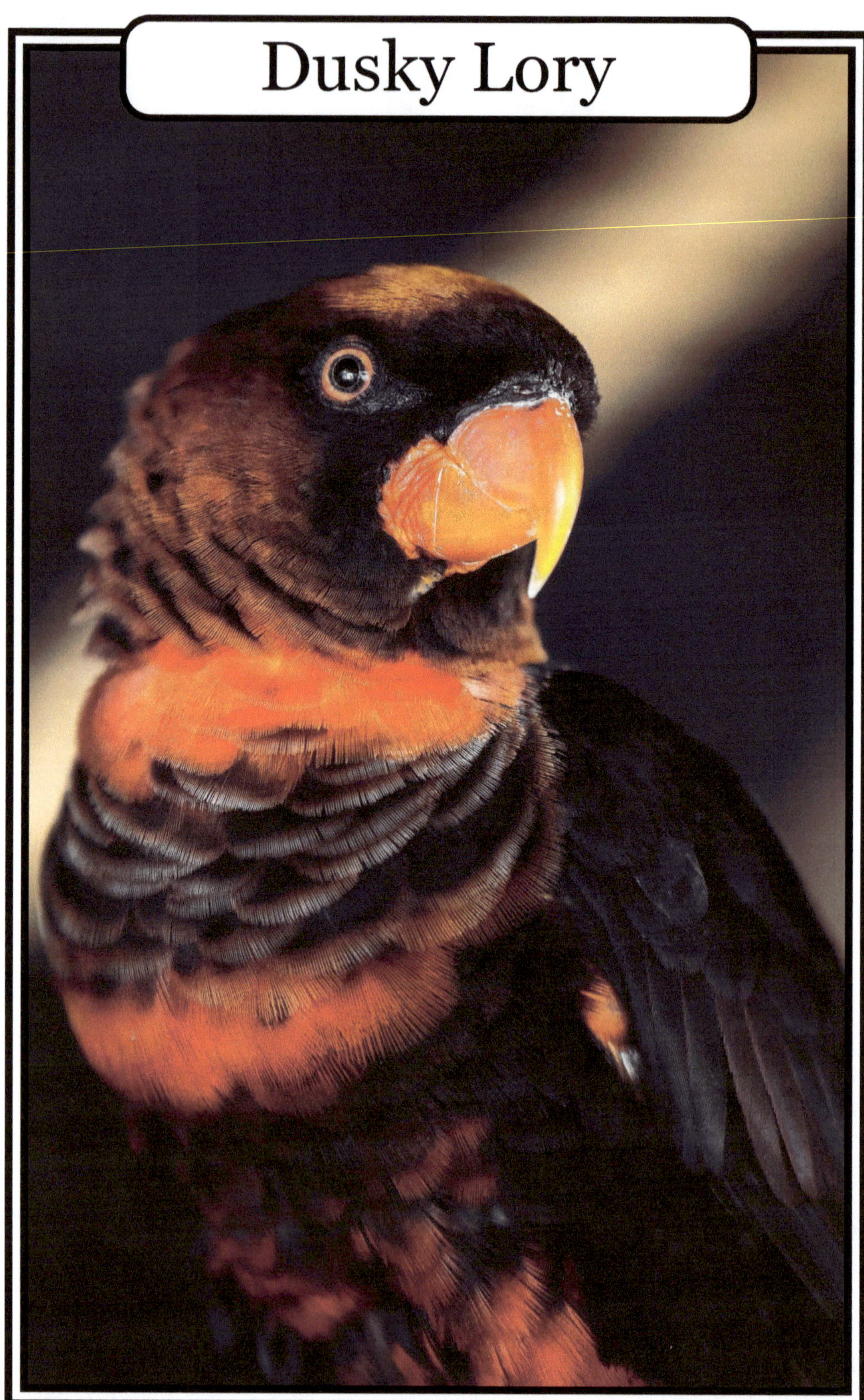

Crimson Finch

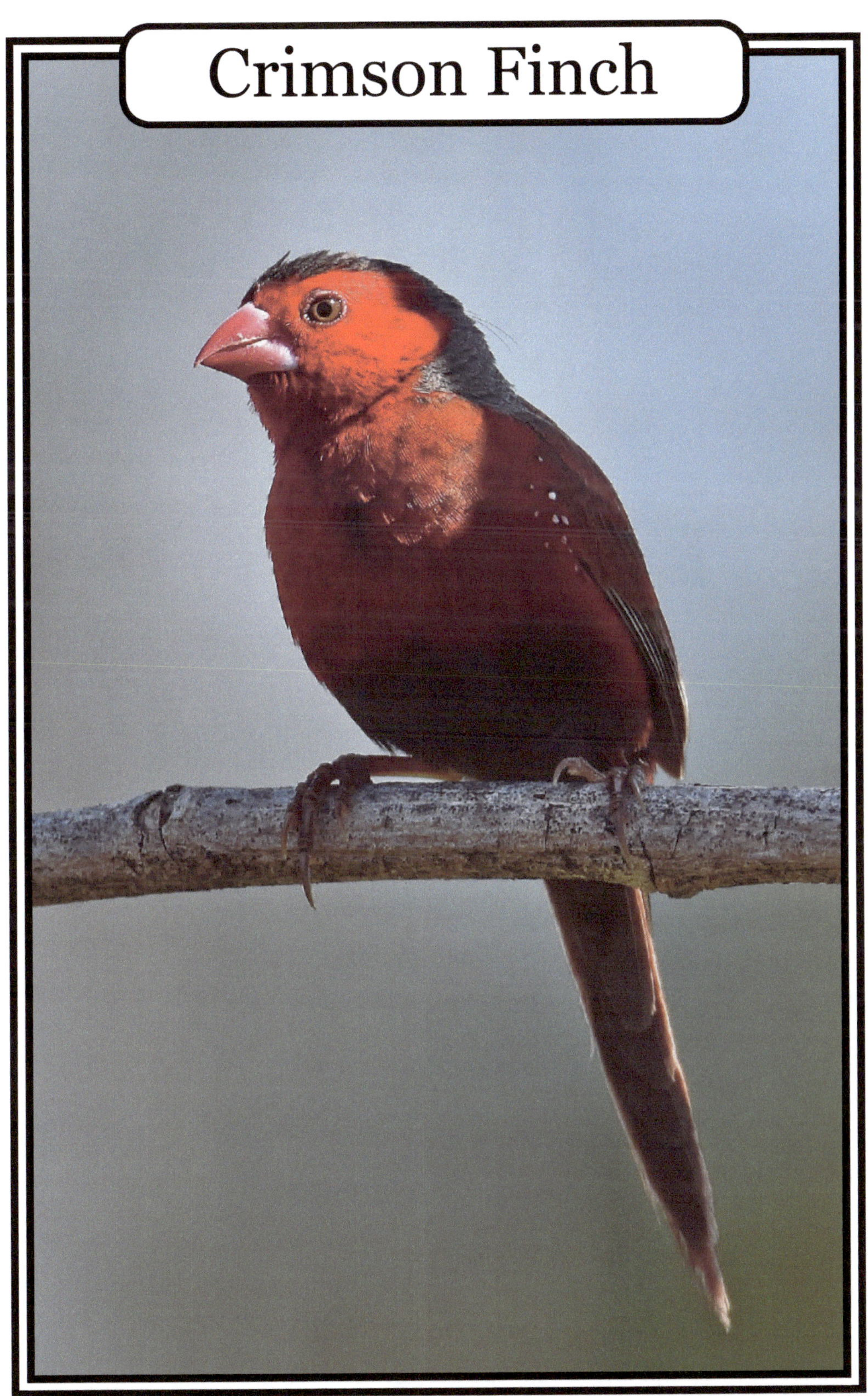

European Goldfinch

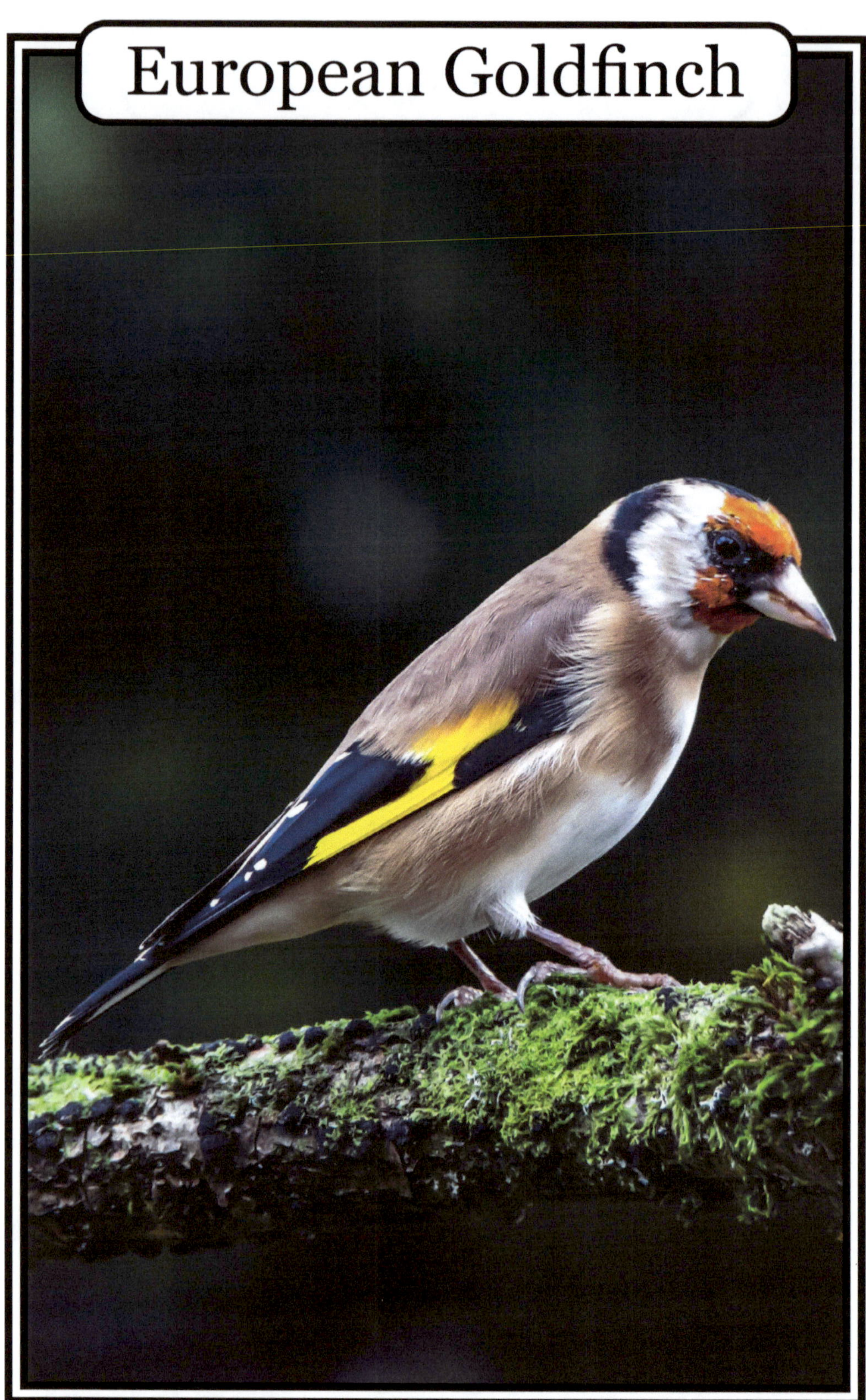

Golden Pheasant

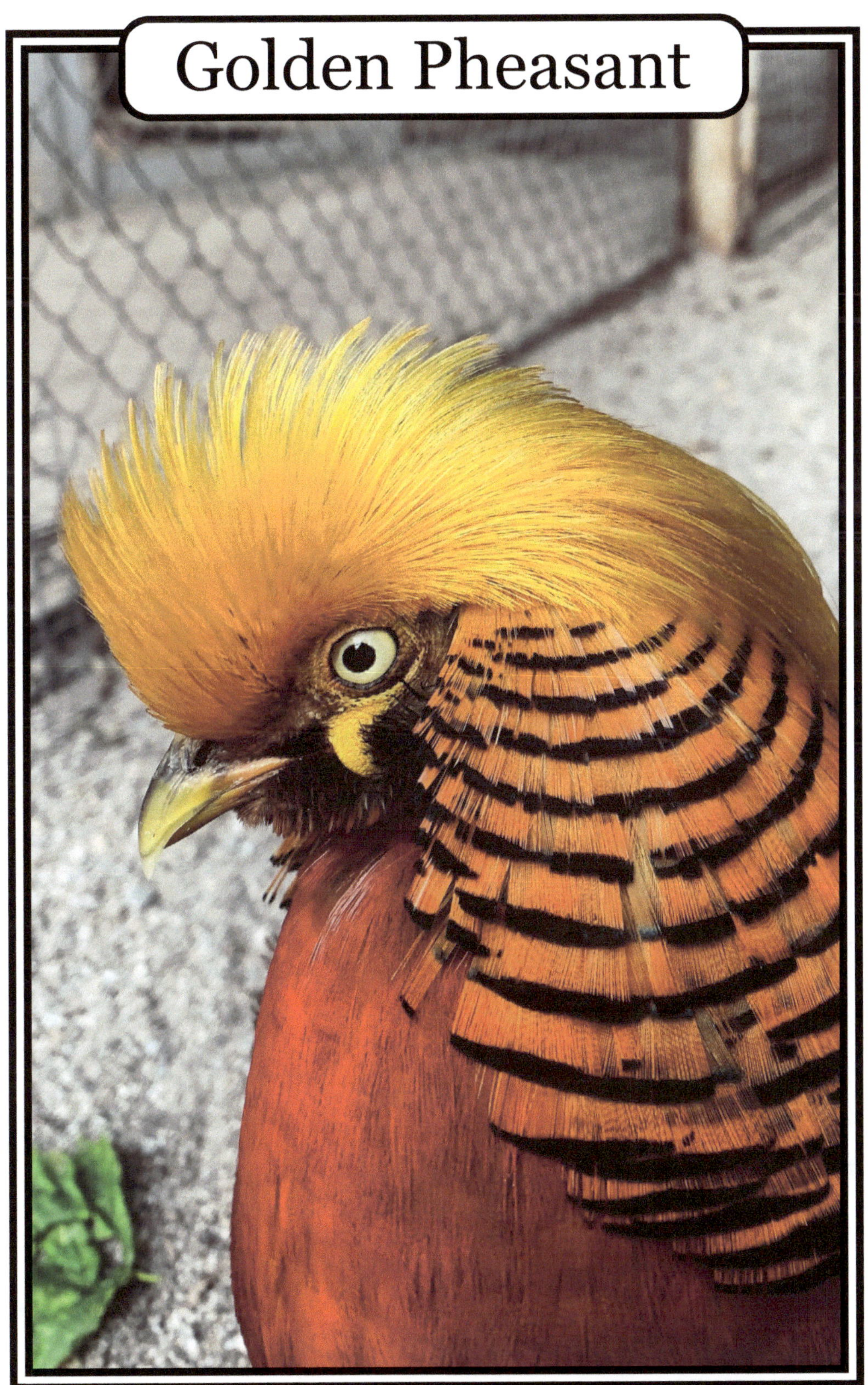

Indigo Bunting

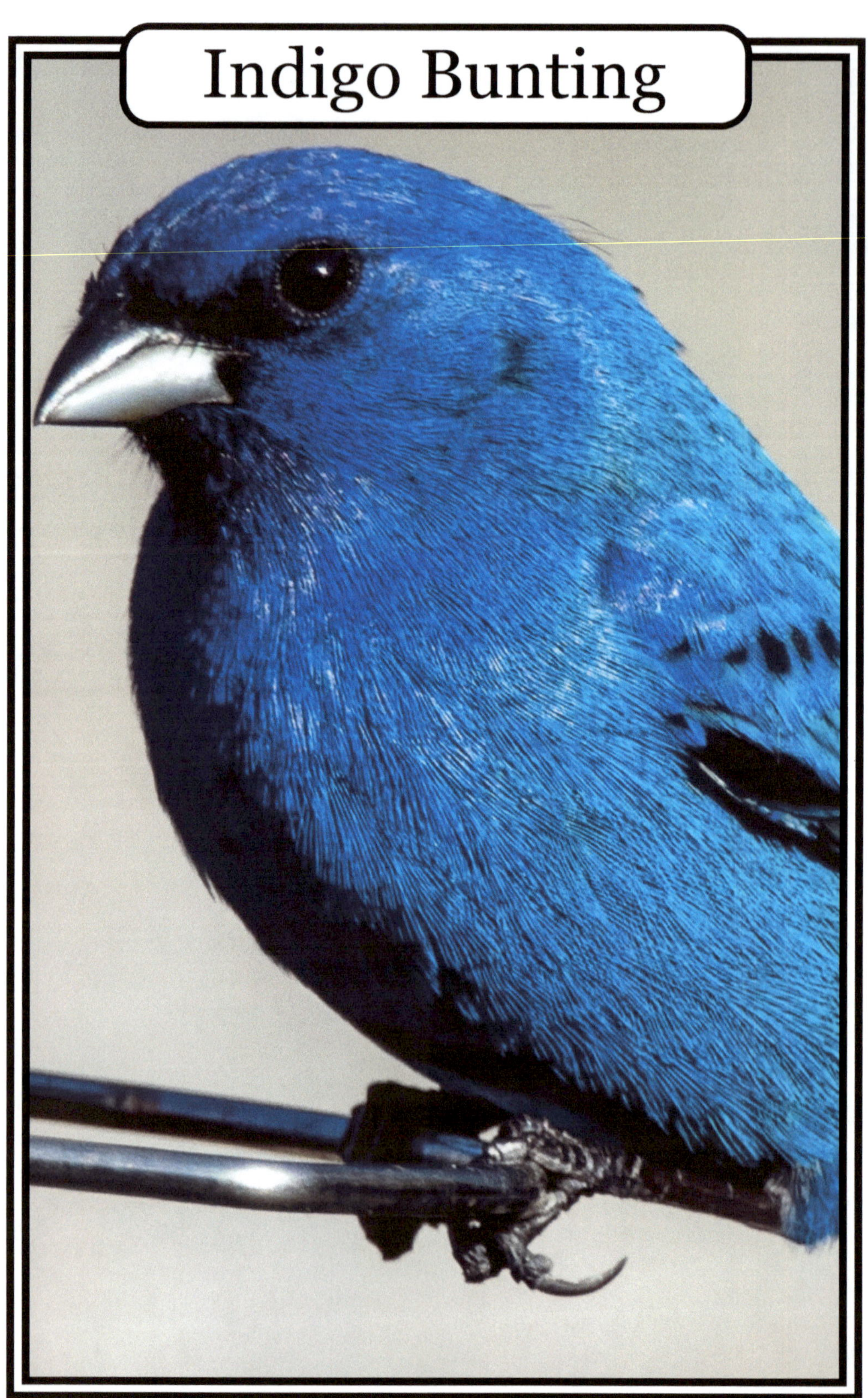

European Roller

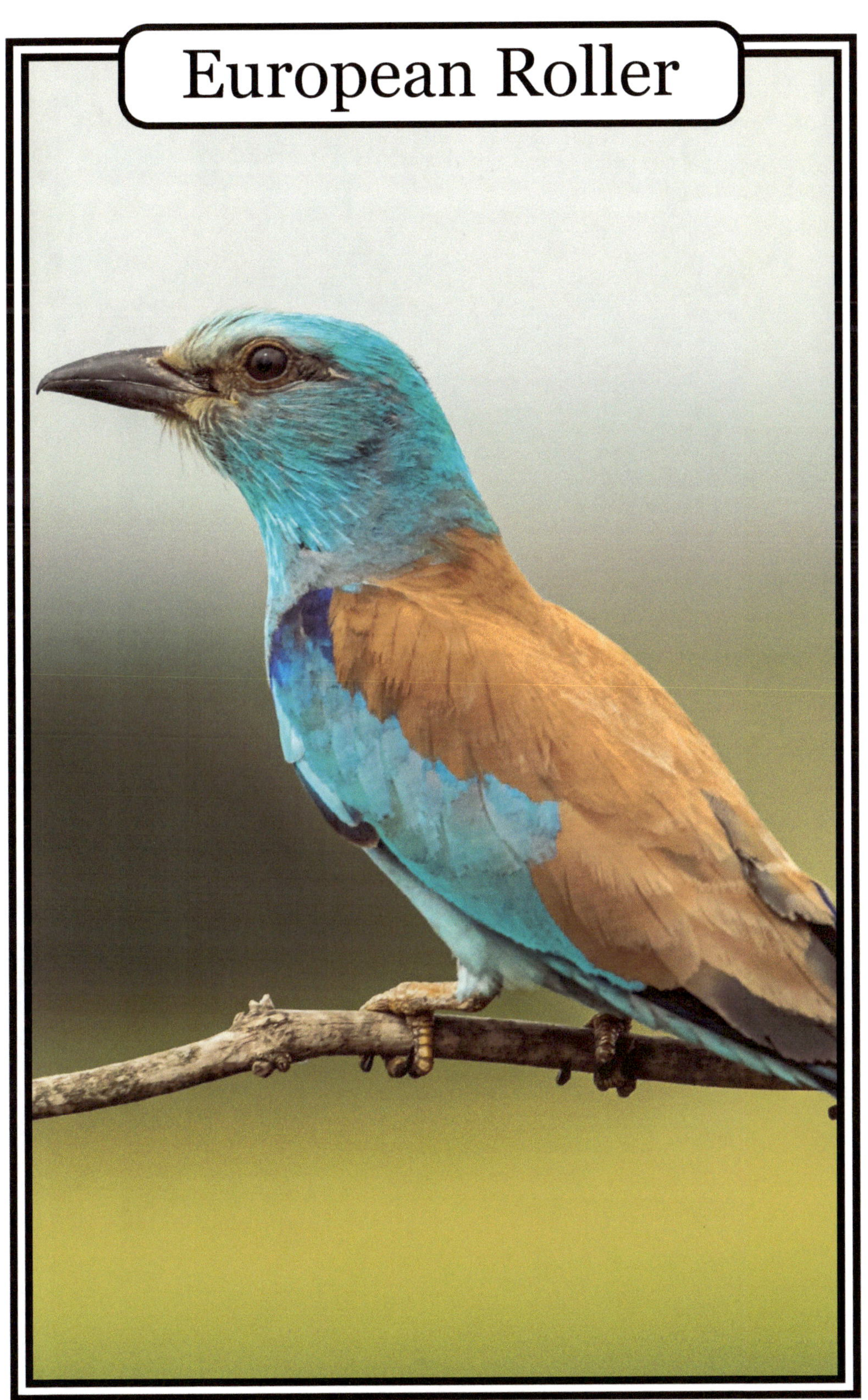

Lilac Breasted Roller

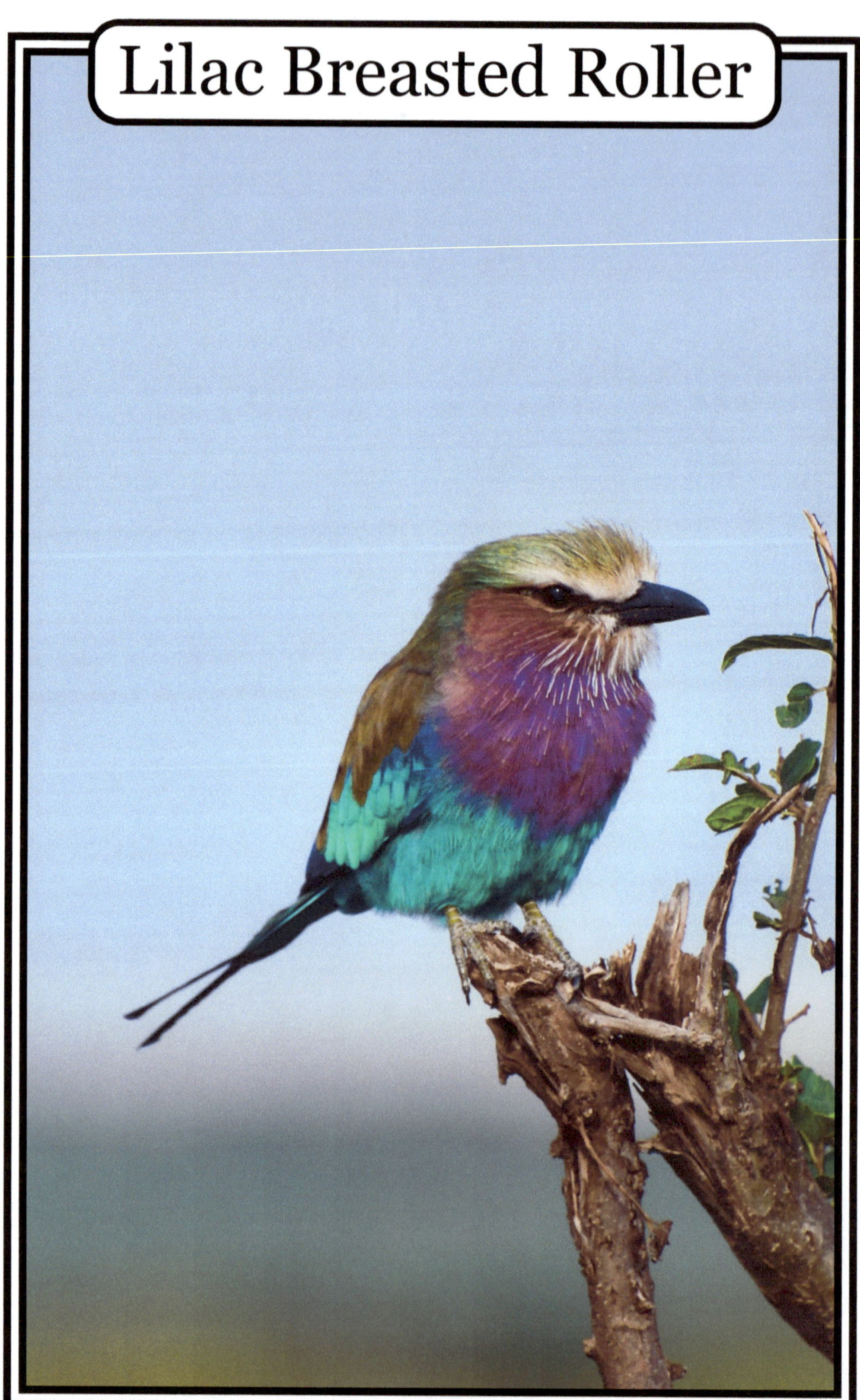

Mandarin Duck

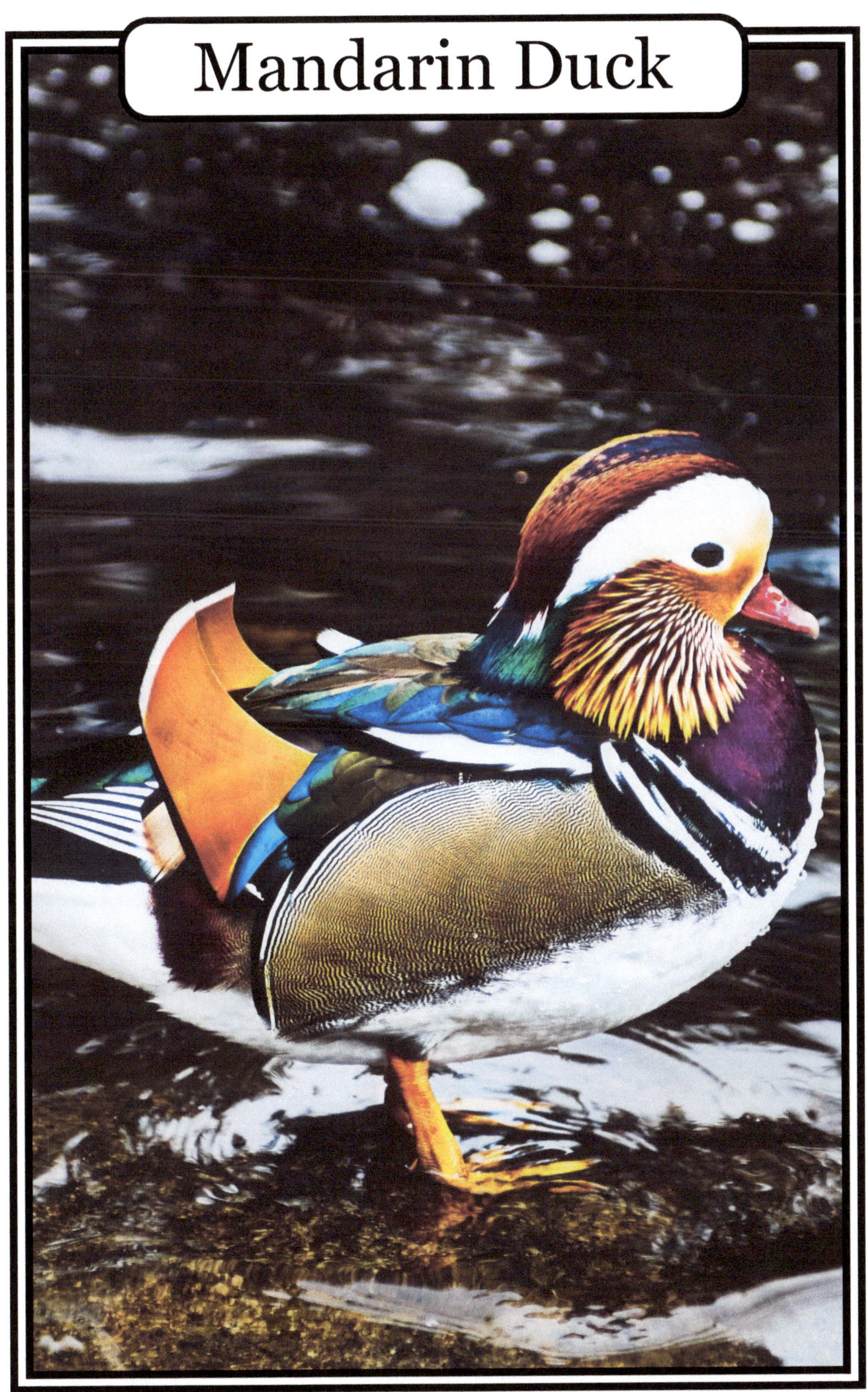

Peacock

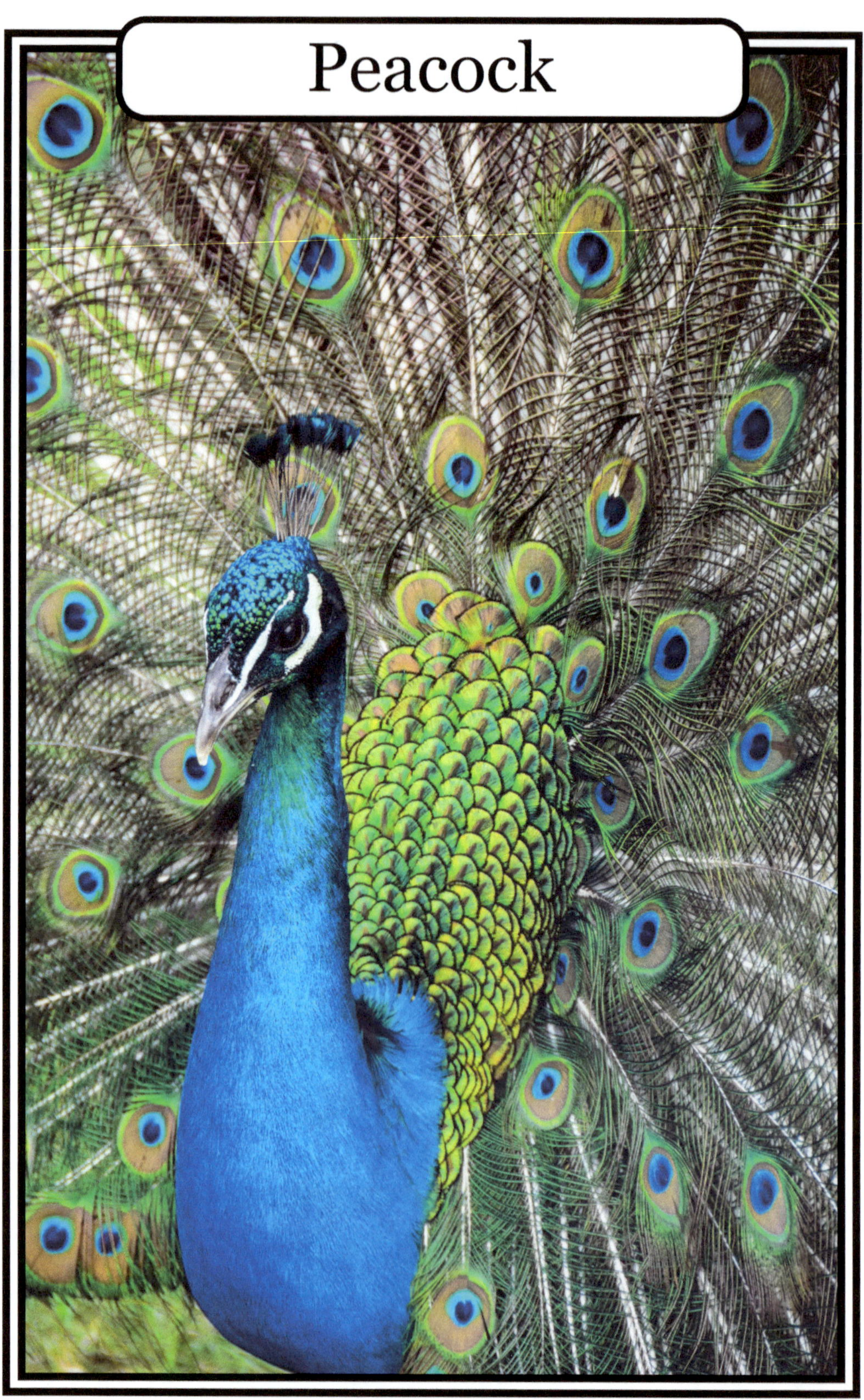

Mallard

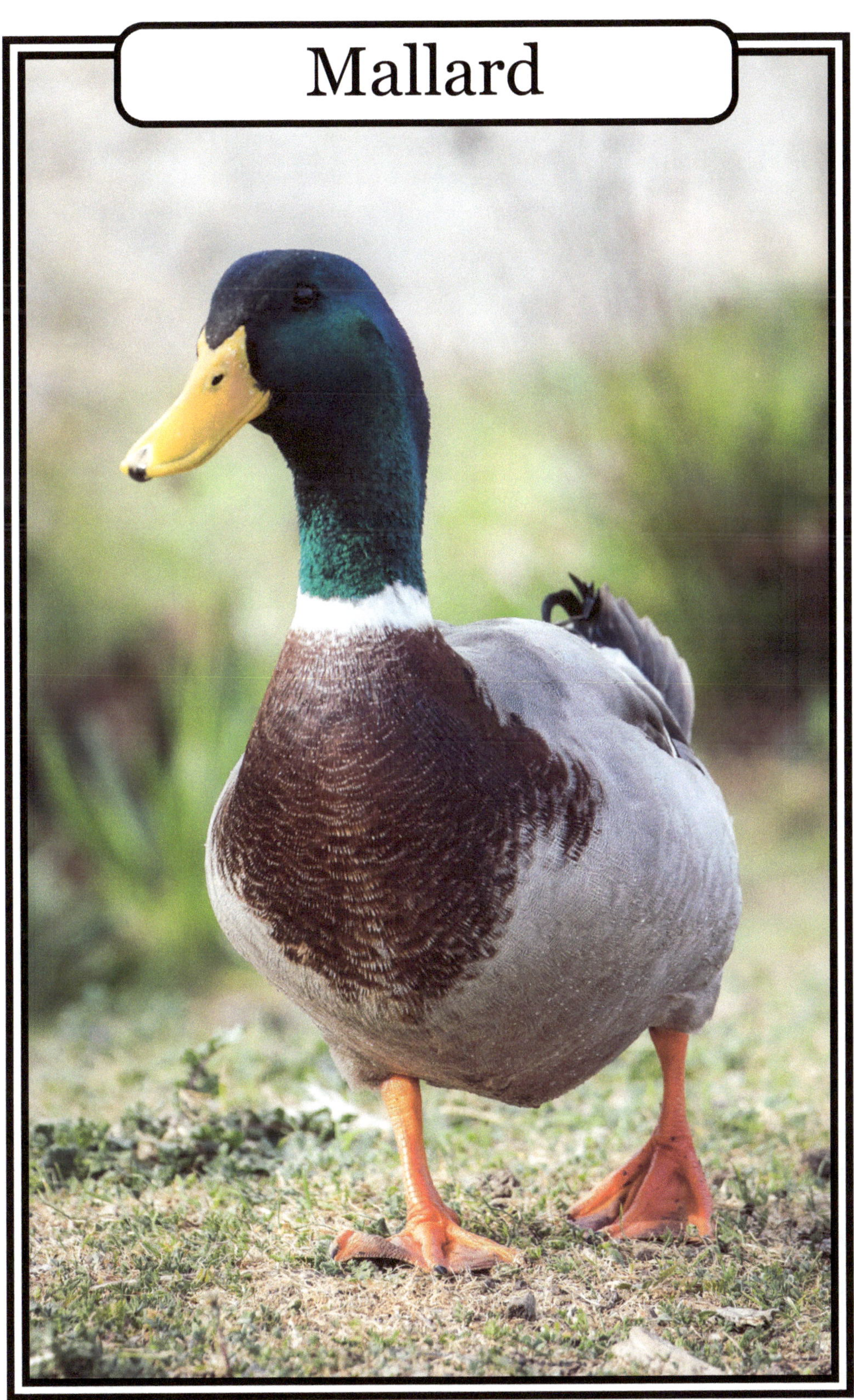

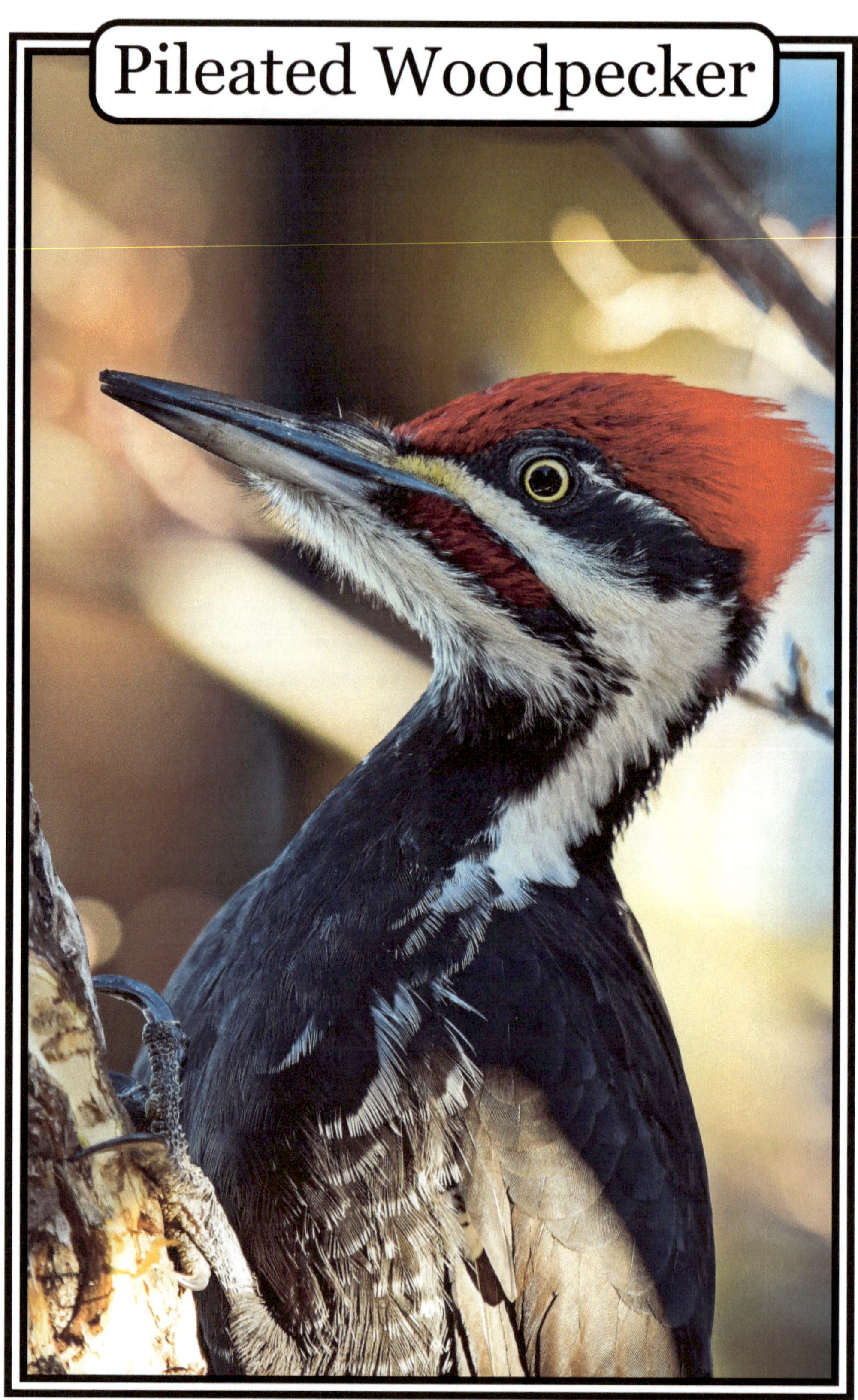
Pileated Woodpecker

Pink Cockatoo

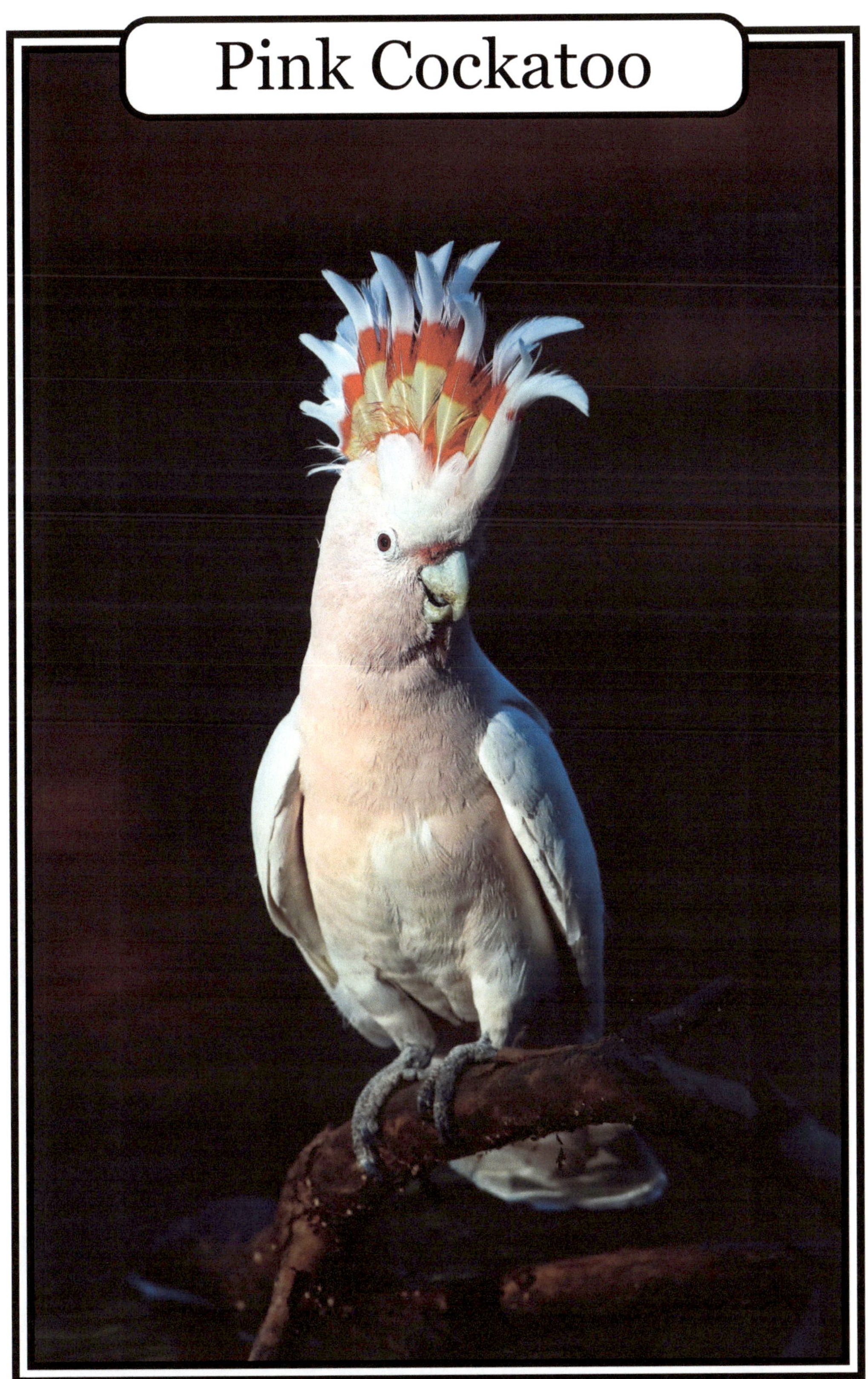

Rainbow Finch

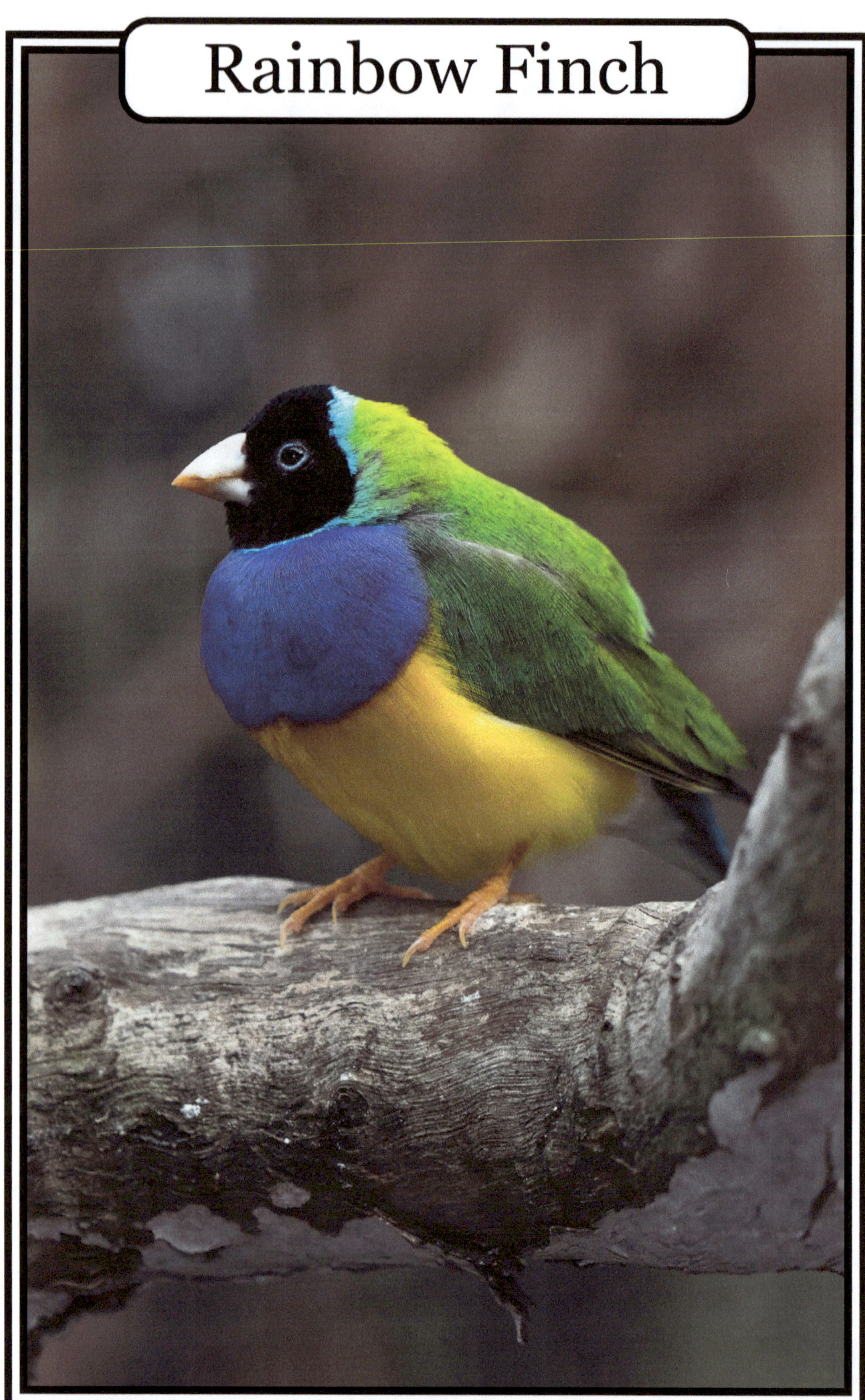

Rainbow Lorikeet

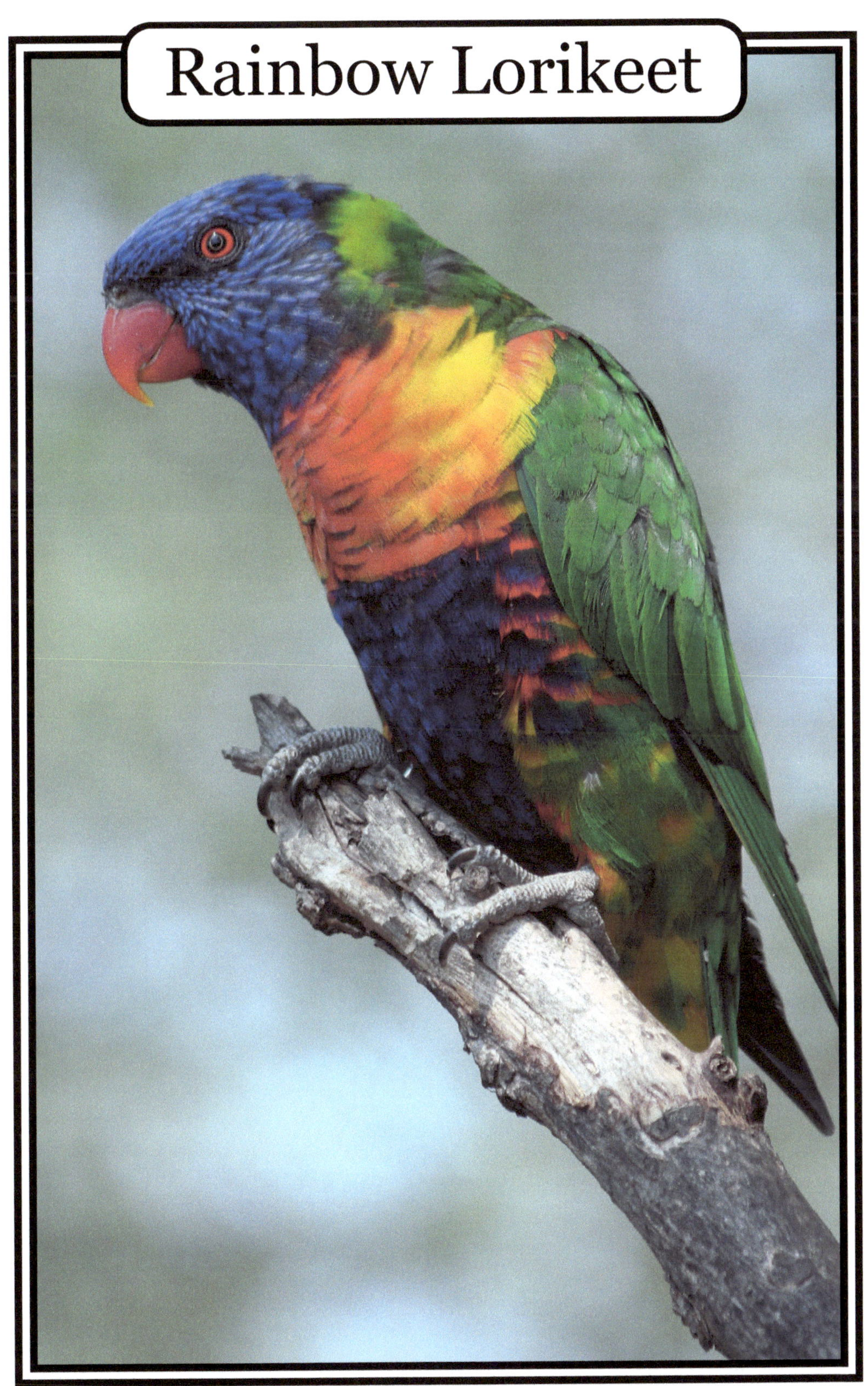

Rose-Ringed Parakeet

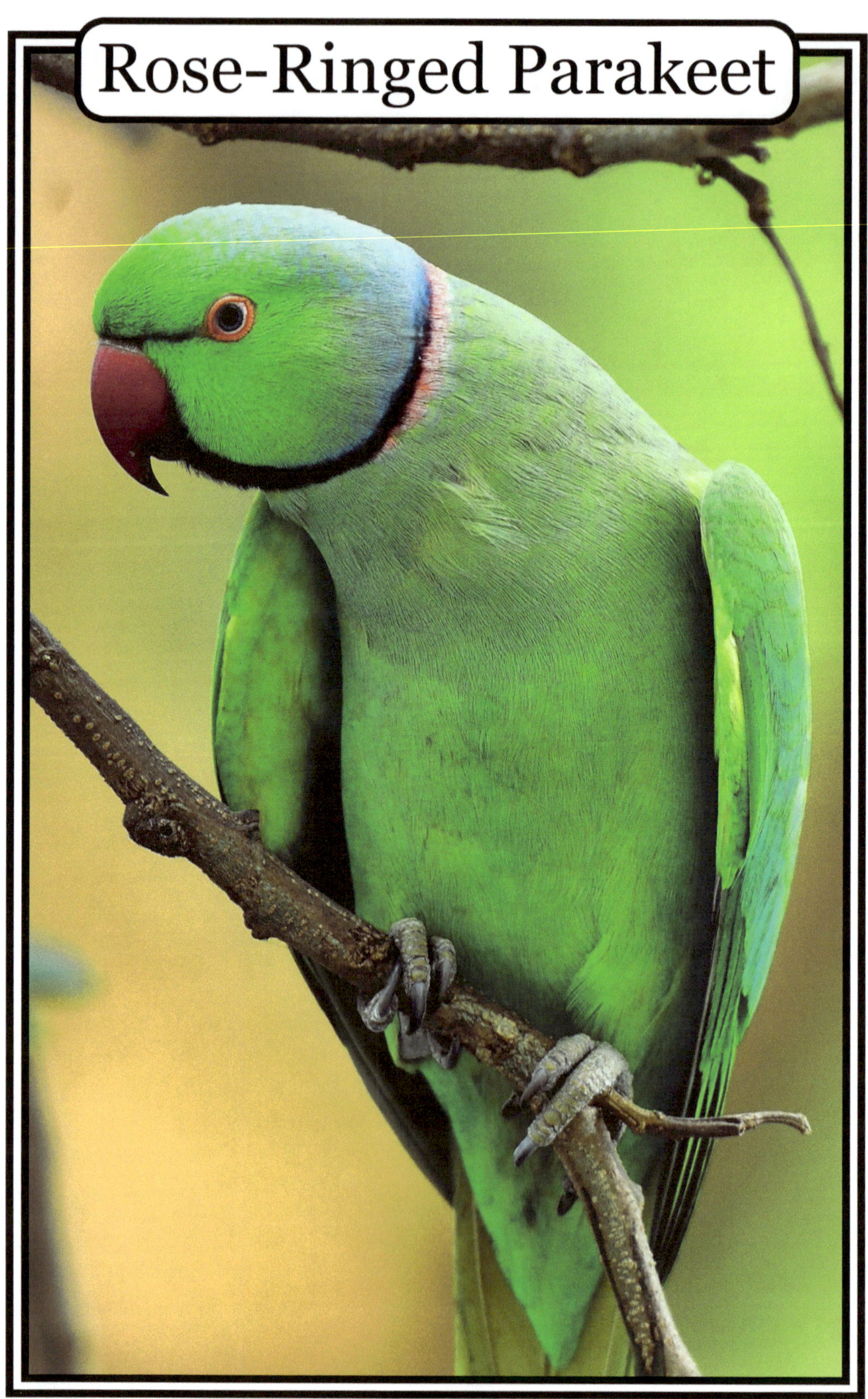

Roseate Spoonbill

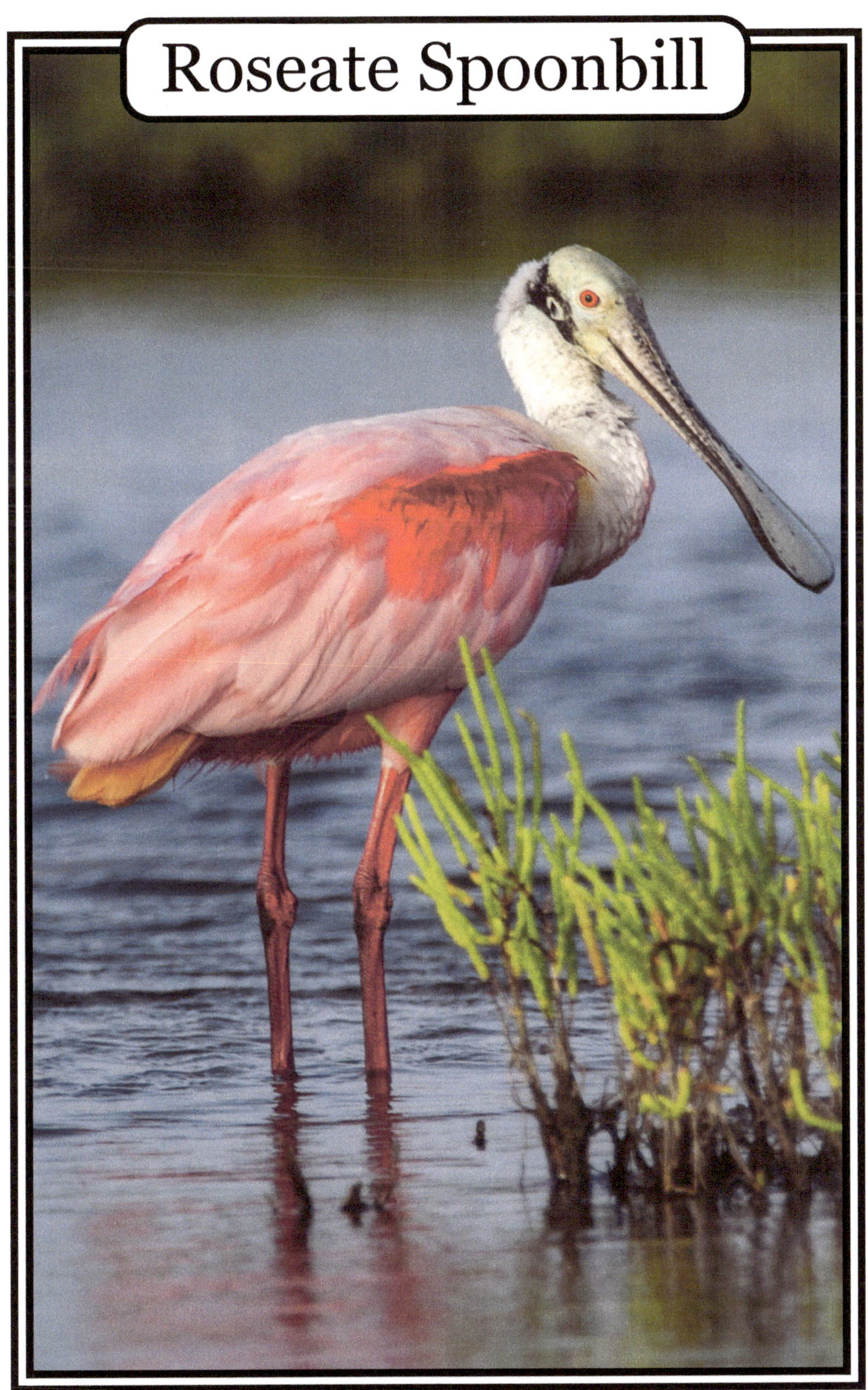

Rosy-Faced Lovebird

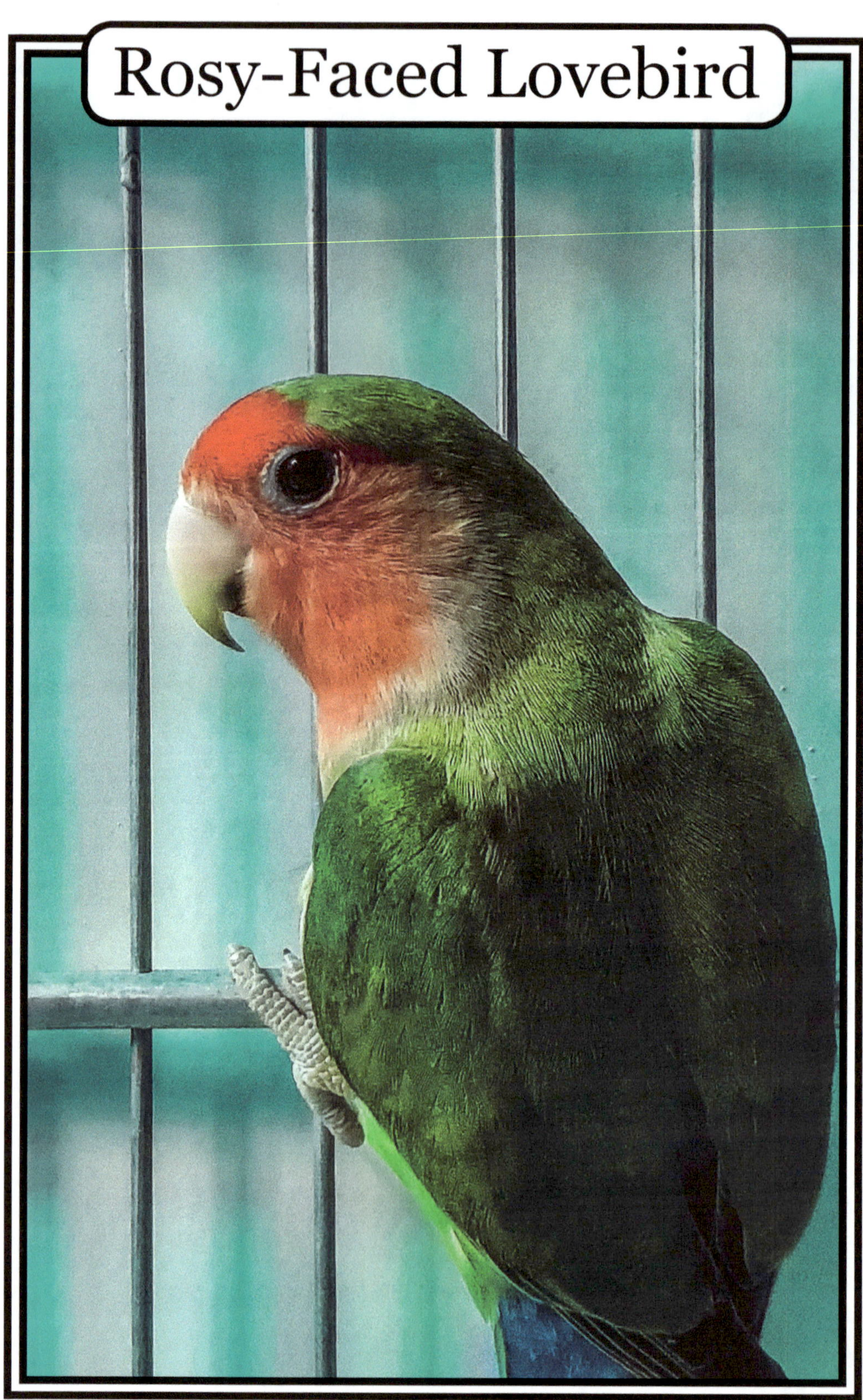

Saddle-Billed Stork

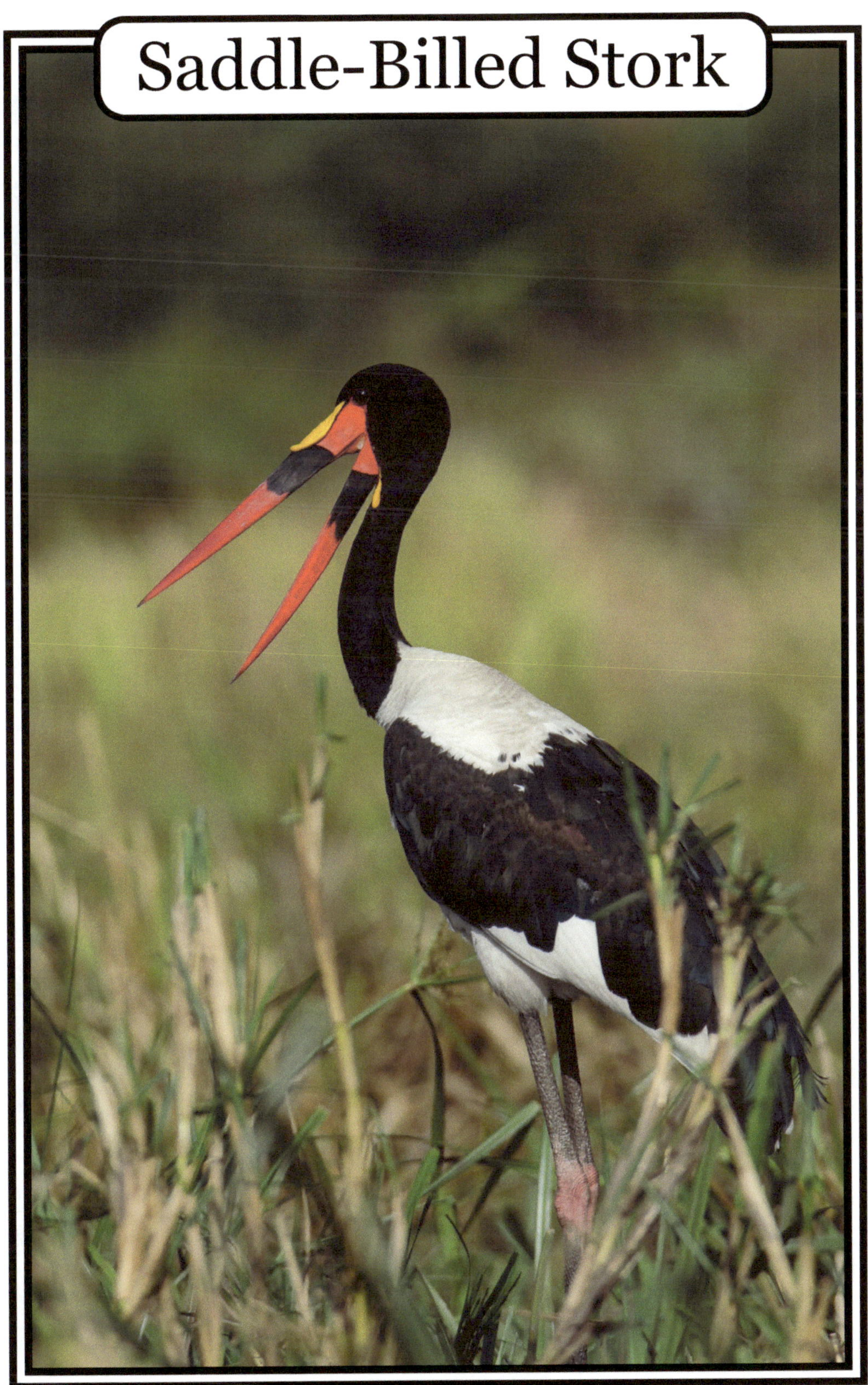

Scarlet Macaw

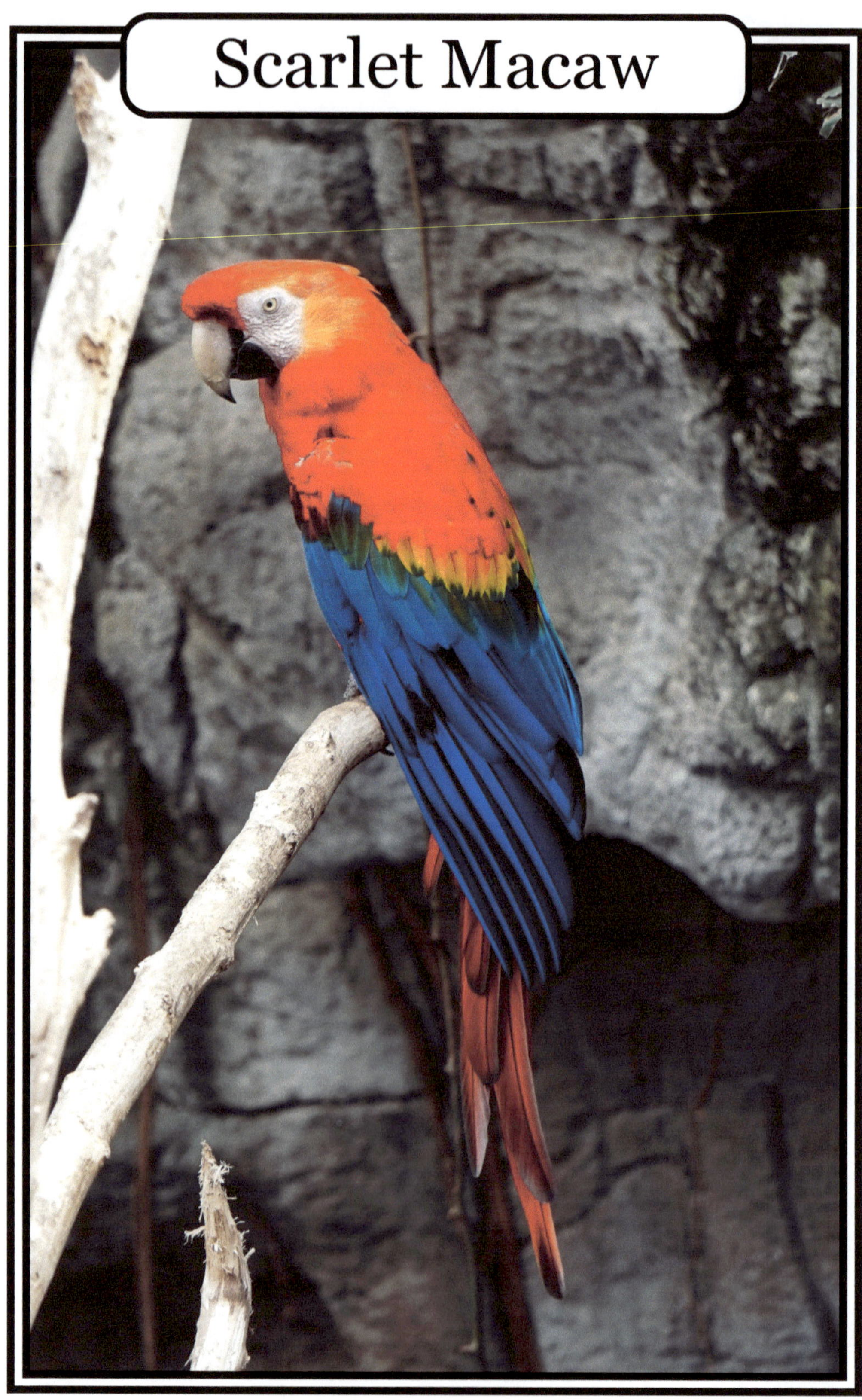

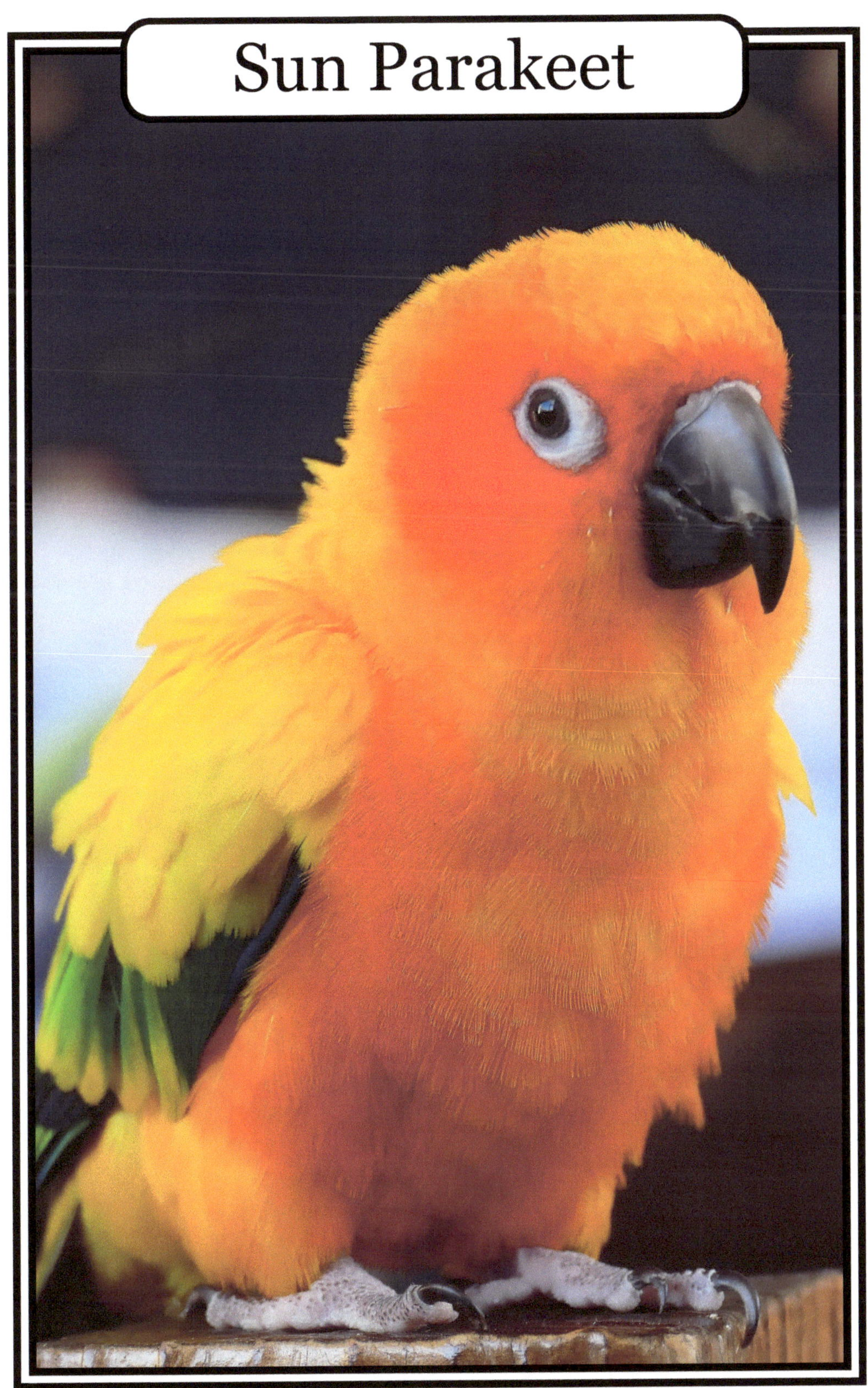# Sun Parakeet

Toco Toucan

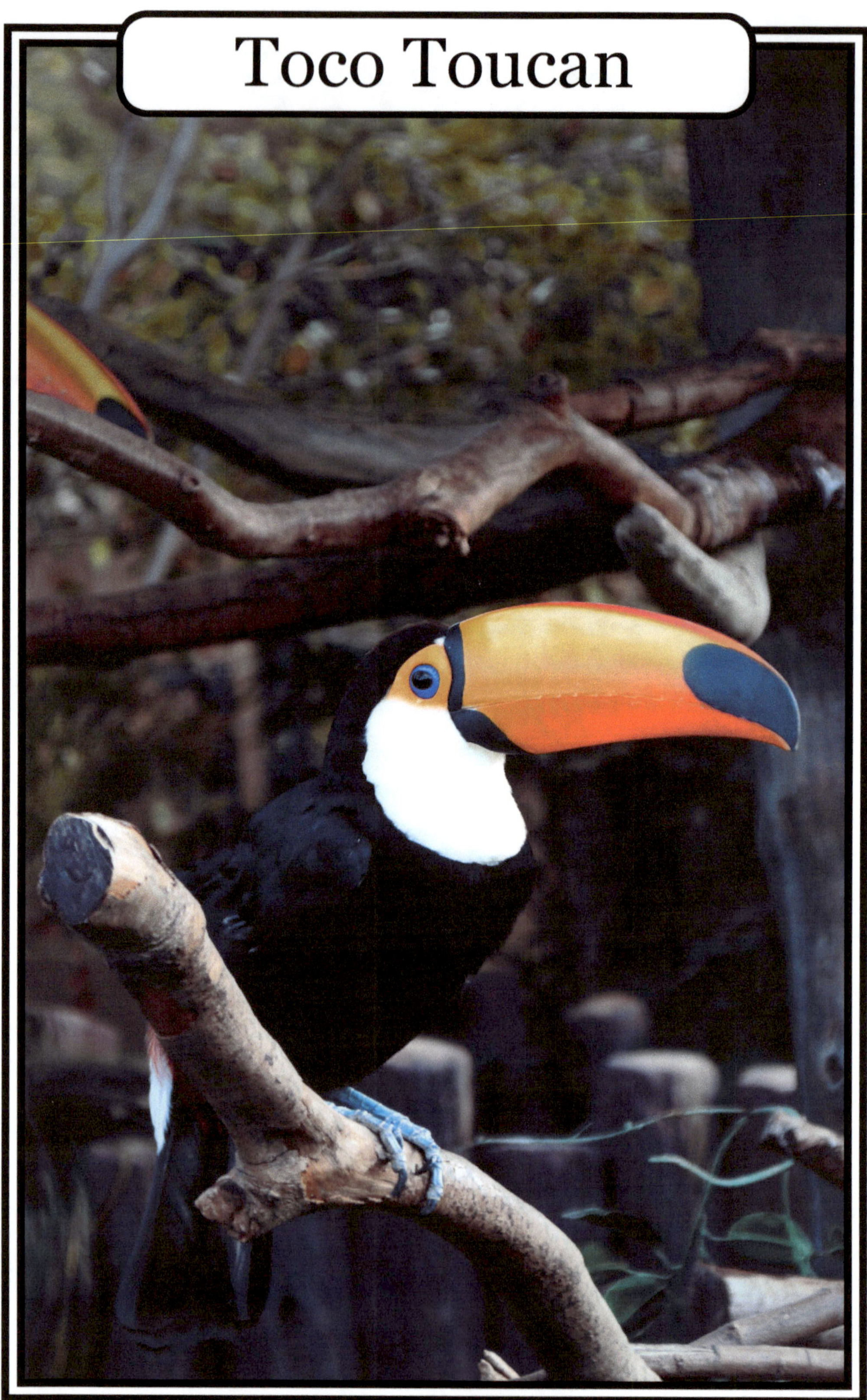

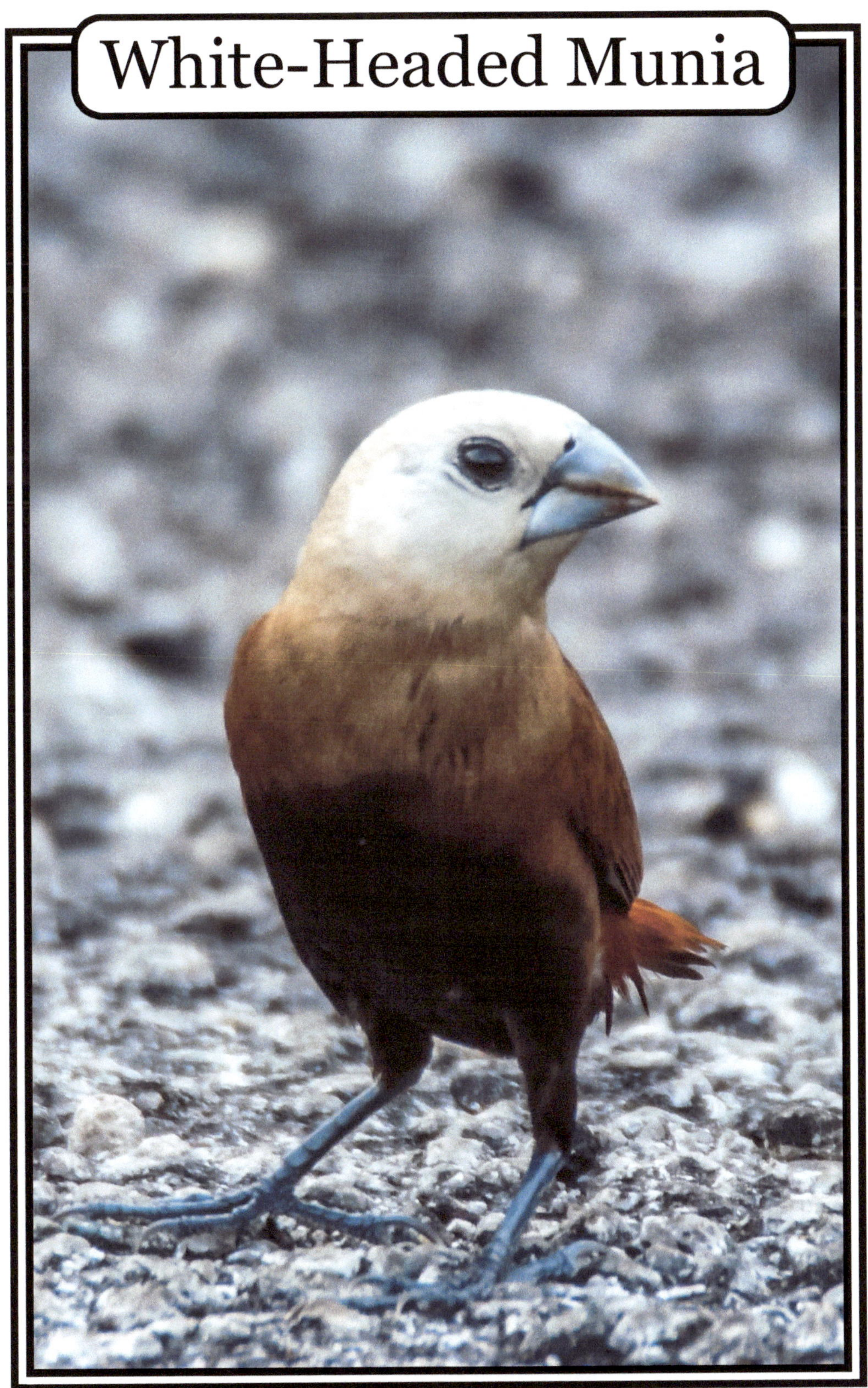

White-Headed Munia

White-Throated Kingfisher

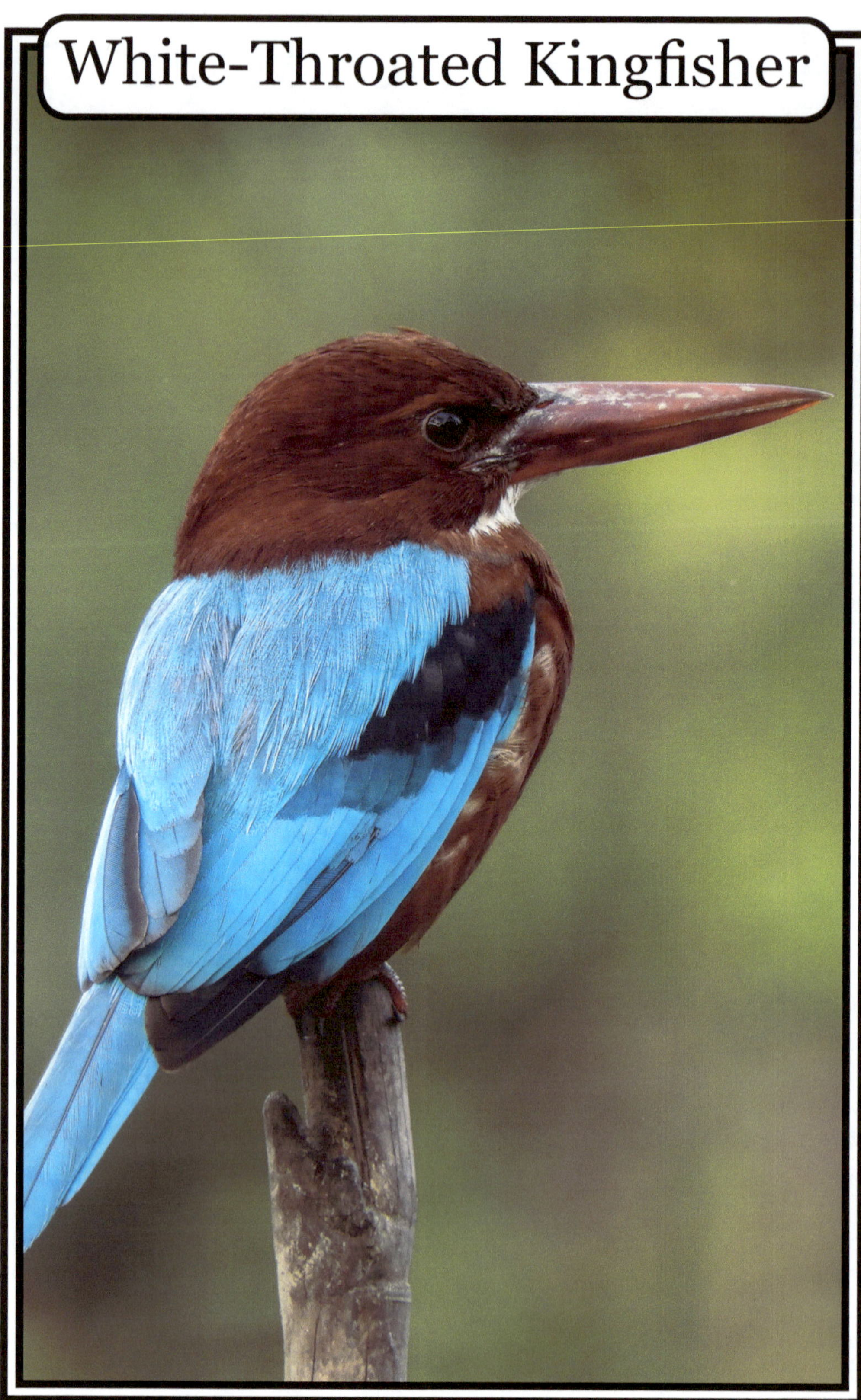

European Starling

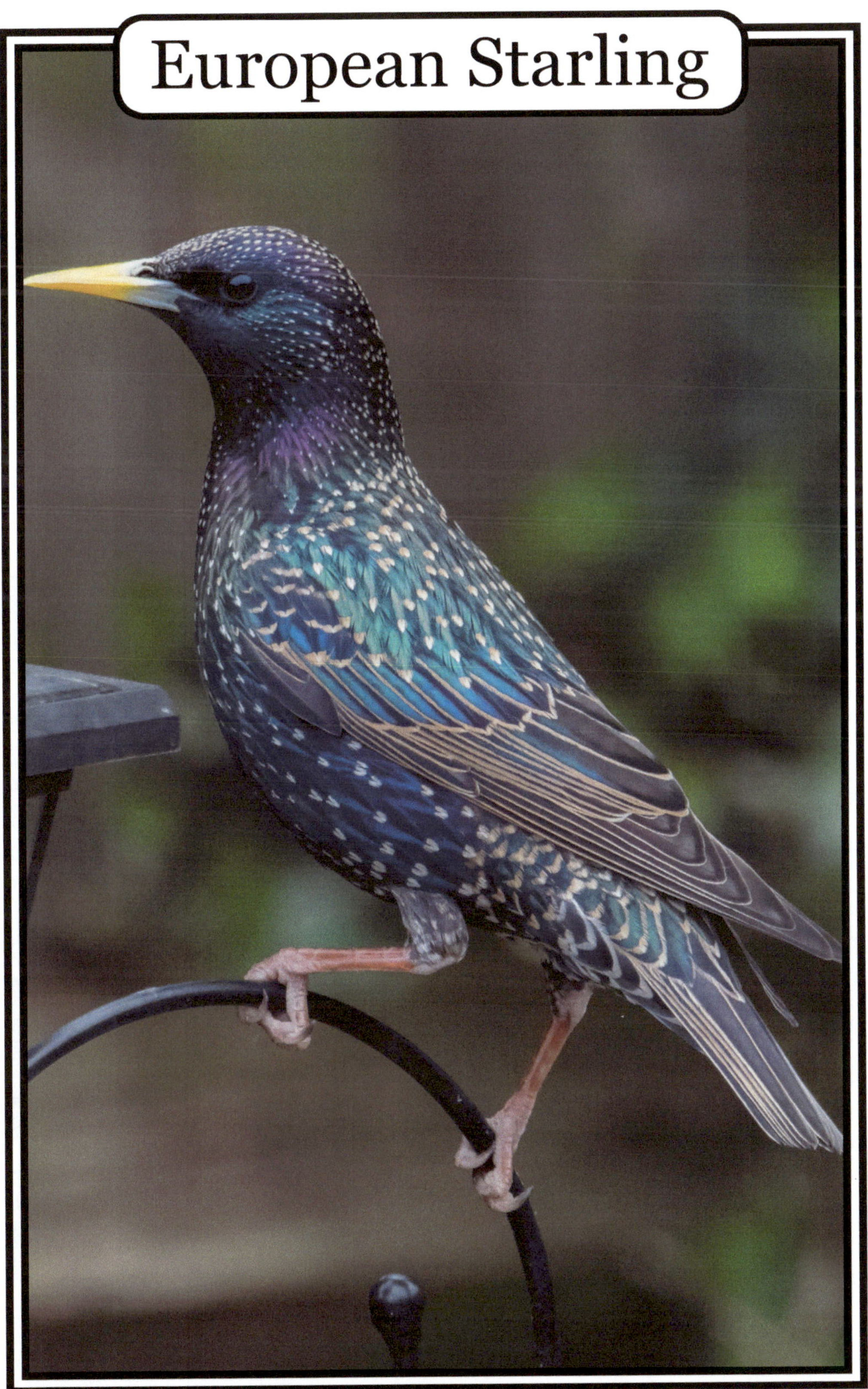

Zebra Finch

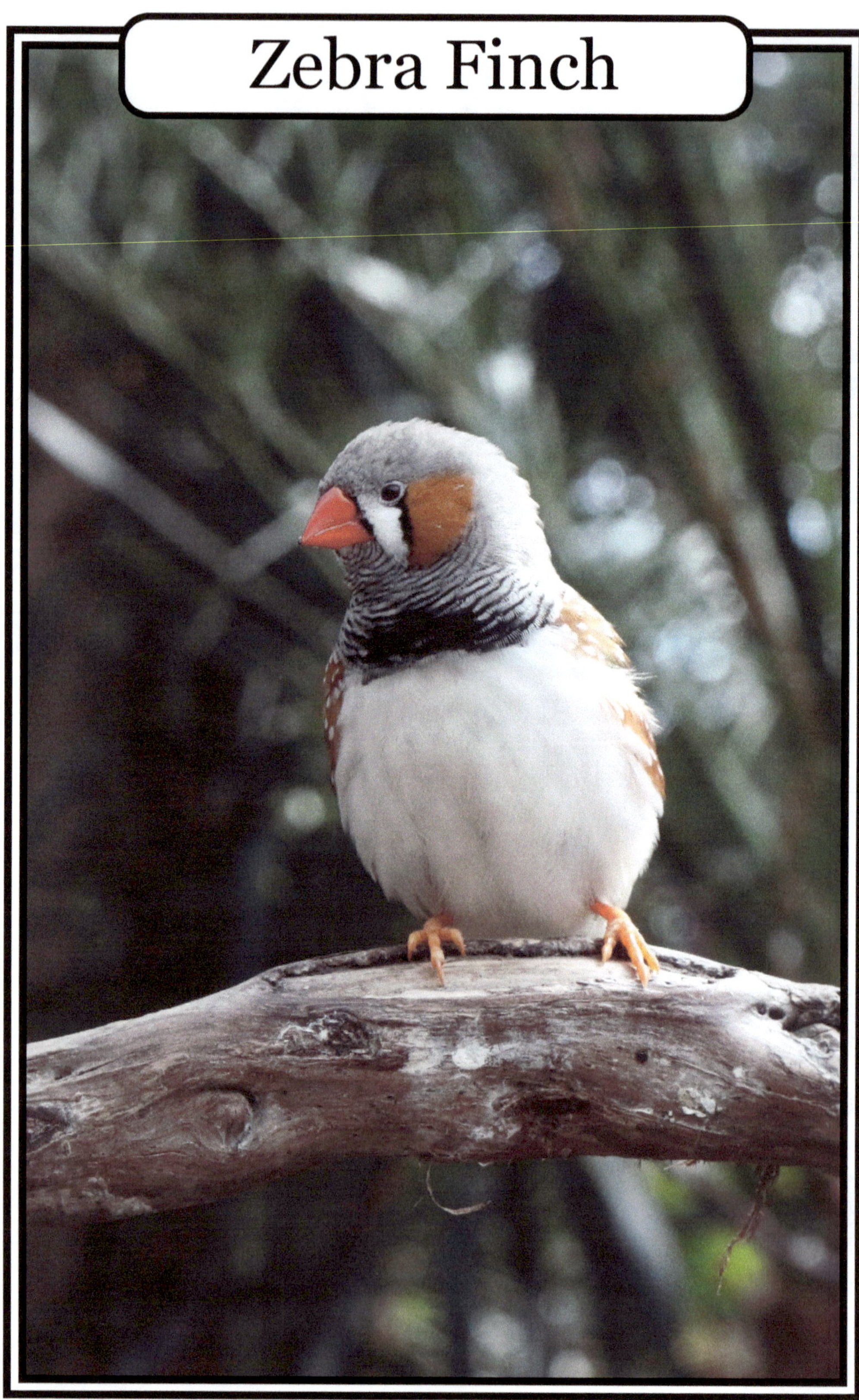

Mountain Bluebird

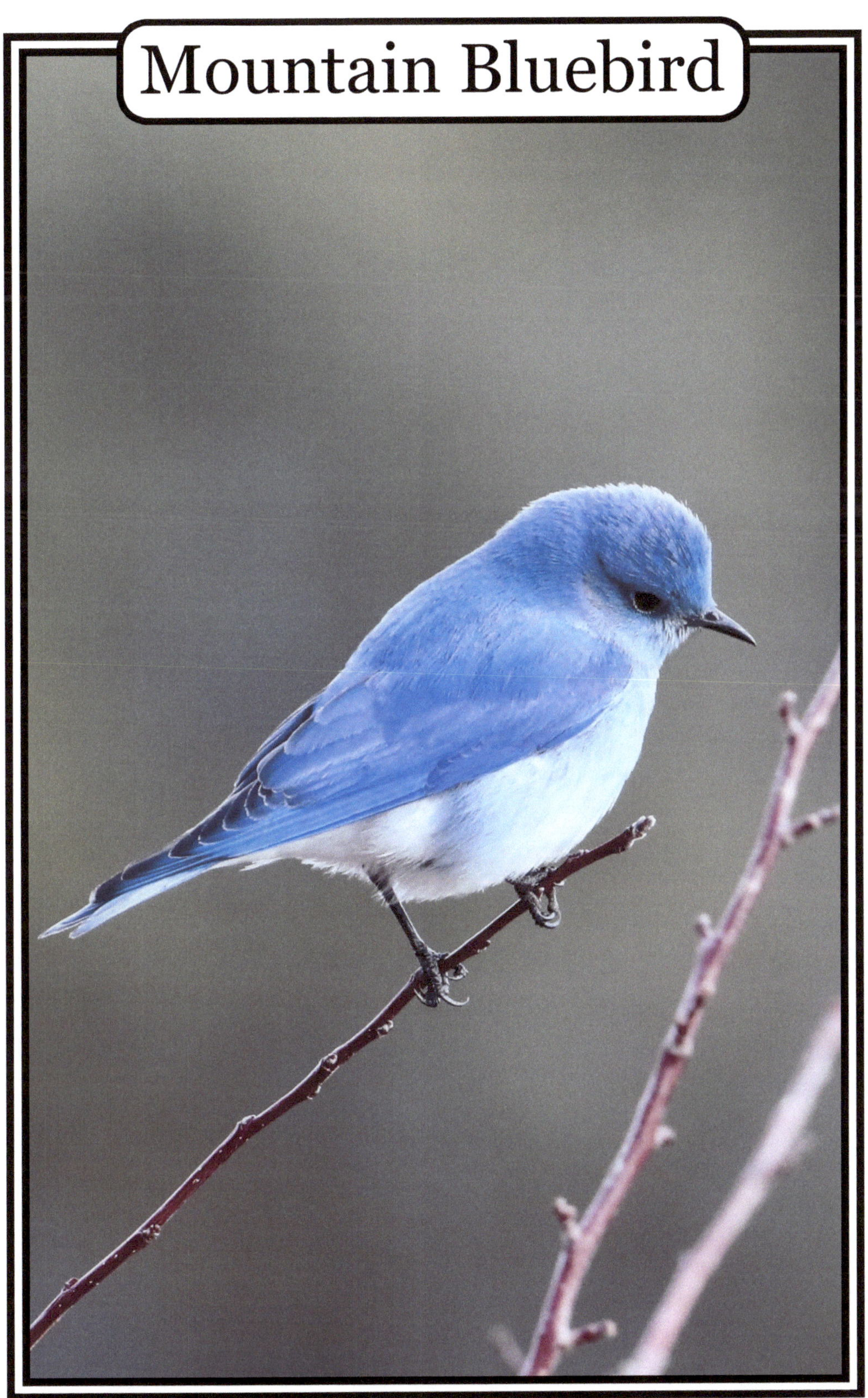

Grey Crowned Crane

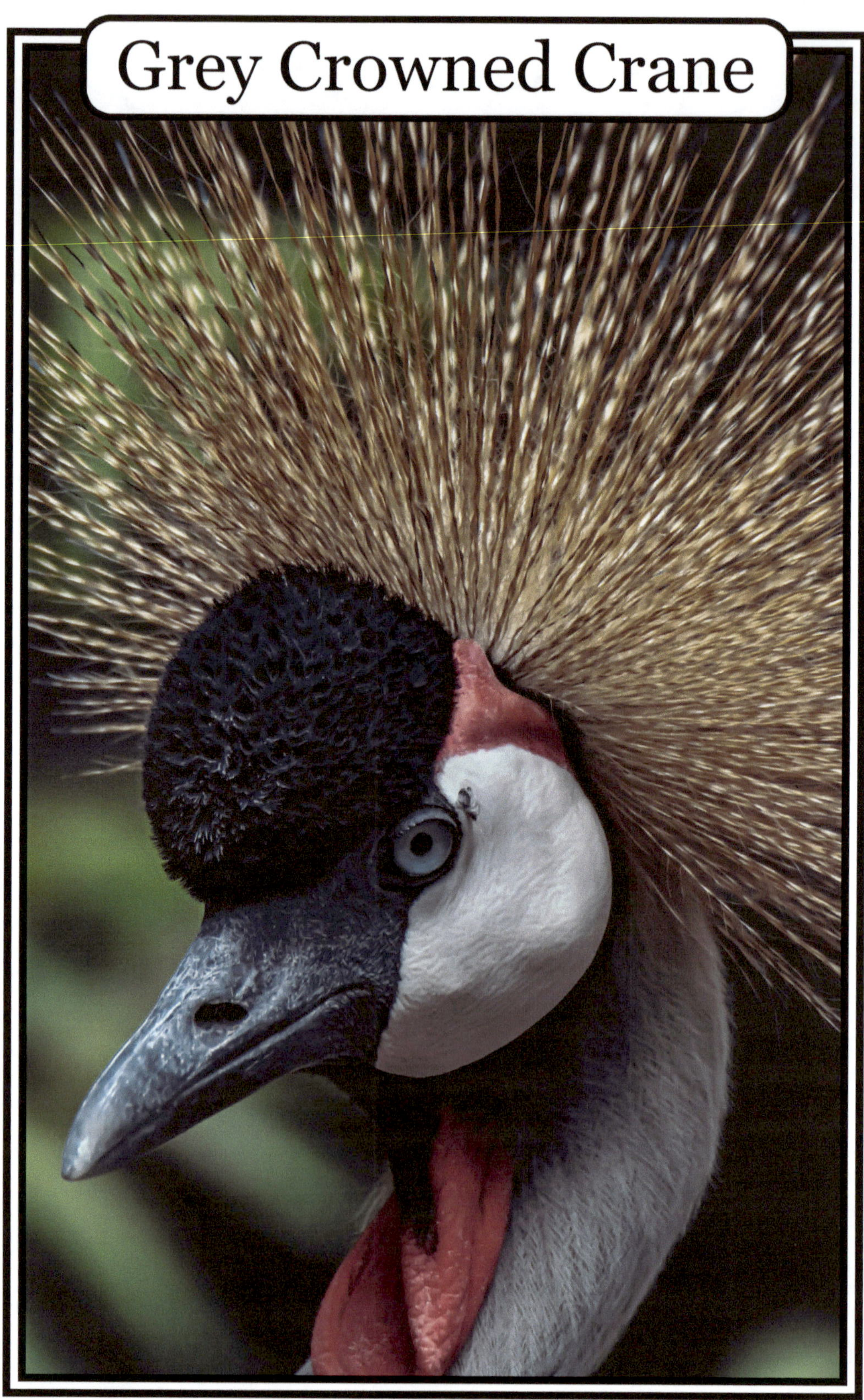

Galah

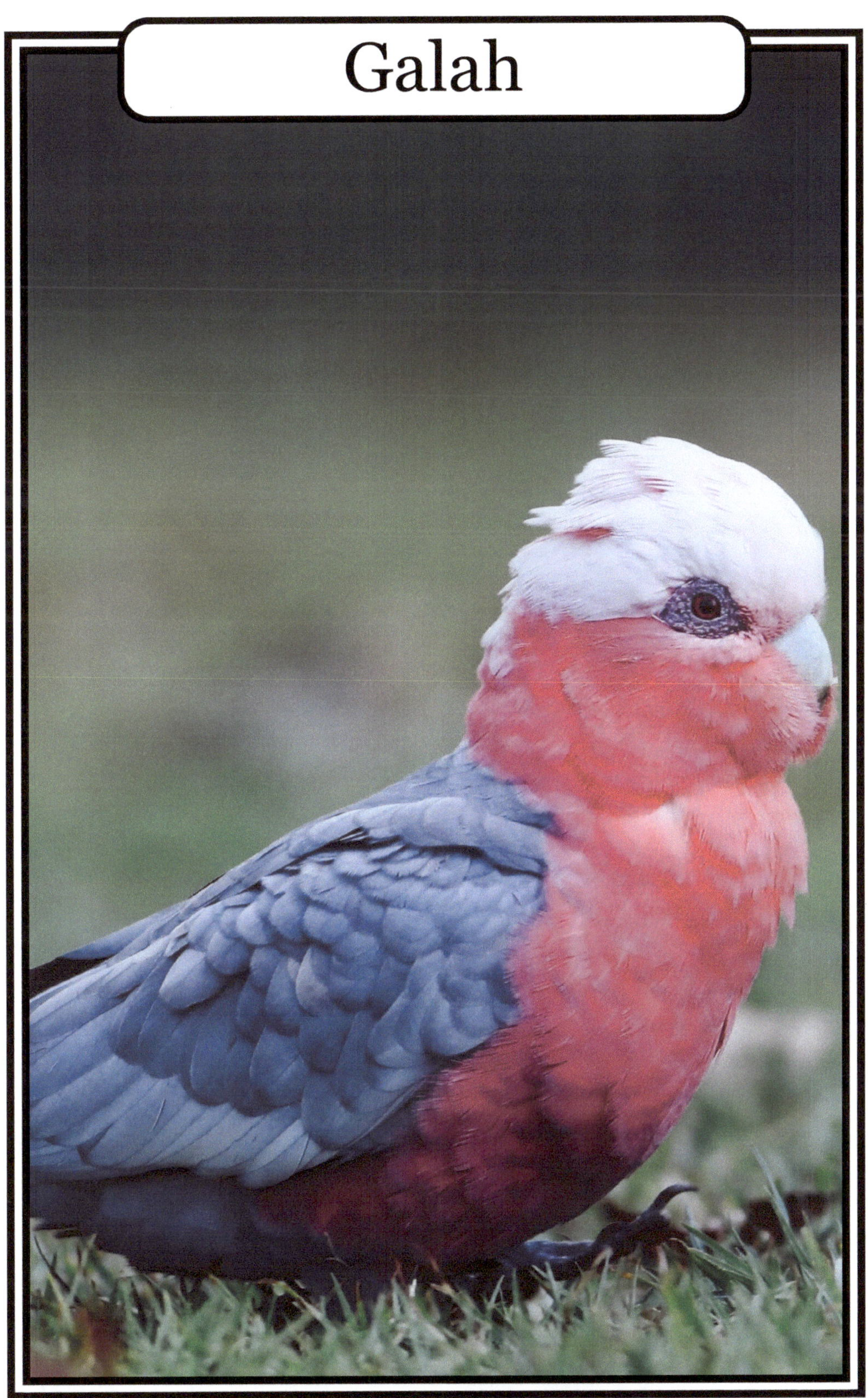

www.ingramcontent.com/pod-product-compliance
Lightning Source LLC
Chambersburg PA
CBHW040947110726
48006CB00007B/1296